Medicine of the Gods

Medicine of the Gods

Basic principles of Âyurvedic medicine

Chris Morgan

© Chris Morgan and Mandrake *of Oxford* 1994 & 02
Second edition

All rights reserved. No part of this work may be reproduced, stored in a retrieval system, or transmitted in any form or by any means, electronic, mechanical, photocopying, recording or otherwise without the prior permission of the publisher.

Mandrake of Oxford
PO Box 250
Oxford, Ox1 1AP
Britain
ISBN 1 869928 37 7

A CIP catalogue record for this book is available from the British Library.

Dedicated to my parents

Printed & bound by Antony Rowe Ltd, Eastbourne

Contents

1 Introduction 9
Ayurveda and the West 11
Another Way of Seeing 12
The Basis of Life 12
The 'Five Elements' (pañcamahâbhûta) 16
The Gunas: Three Strands of the Mind 19
The Tissues of the Body 21

2 Health and the Origin of Disease 23
The Three Humour Theory 24
The Ecology of the Humours 28
The Indian Seasons and the Cycle of Humours and Tastes 30
Possible European Cycle of Humours and Tastes 31
The Functions of the Three Humours 35

3 Temperament and Constitution 37
The Unctuous or Watery Type
    (shlesmala or kaphaja) 38
The Fiery Type (pittala) 39
The Air Type (vataja) 40
Mental Temperament 42

4 Common diseases of Ayurvedic medicine and their ancient antecedents 47
Diseases of the Vedic 'system' 50
I. The Yákshma/Takmán Complex of Diseases 50
1. Yákshma *50*

2. Jâyânya 53
3. Kshetriyá 53
4. Rápas (Disease) 54
5. Hriddyotá, Harimán 54
6. Balâsa (swellings).. 54
7. Takmán 54
8. Kasa 55

II Other Internal Diseases 55
1. Amîvâ 55
2. Víshkandha-Sámskandha 55
3. Udára (Dropsy) 56
4. Únmadita and únmatta 56
5. Krími:17 (Worms) 56
6. (Urine retention) 57

III External Diseases 57
1. (Fractures) 57
2. Haemorrhage, especially menorrhagia21 57
3. Skin disorders 58
The New Diseases of Ayurvedic Times 59
Ayurvedic diseases and their possible social significance 59
1. Shosha (Consumption) 59
2. Diabetes (Prameha) 63
Modern Data on Diabetes 66
3. Tumours & Cysts 67
4. Leprosy (Hansen's Disease) 68
5. Epilepsy 70
6. Piles 70
7. Renal Calculus 71
Conclusion 72

5 Food 75
Sushruta's catalogue of meats 75
Caraka's catalogue of meats 78
Caraka's catalogue of cereals 82
Rationality and ayurvedic medicine 85

The formal analysis of taste 87
The Range of Ayurvedic experience 91
Conclusion 96
Sushruta's catalogue of meats 97
1.JANGALA 97
2. ANÜPA 101
Caraka's catalogue of meats31 104
Endnotes 110

Bibliography **113**
Index **123**

8 *Chris Morgan*

1
Introduction

This book is a study of the Hindu system of medicine known as Âyurveda[1], which has its beginnings in the sixth century BCE[2] and thrives even to the present-day. There was a time when the ideas of Ayurveda were new. Indeed the Ayurvedic physicians seem to be aware of such a fact when compiling their original treatises. There was once a celebrated doctor called Caraka—we do not know exactly when he lived—it is presumed to be in the second century of the present era. He was one of the greatest physicians that has ever lived. Caraka was very keen to justify his attempt to revise the venerated and almost sacrosanct methods of the older Vedic shaman-physicians. He records the fact that the gods themselves were perplexed by the continued existence of disease, which was a hindrance

---

1 From now on the term Âyurveda will be spelt Ayurveda, i.e. without the diacritic over the a.
2 Stands for 'Before the Common Era' a more modern designation for what used to be termed BC or 'Before Christ.'

to humanity's progress towards enlightenment. These same gods, so he claimed, had prepared the way for Ayurveda to be taught to the human race.[3]

Caraka was being very daring when he suggested that a healthy body is a prerequisite for salvation. Many strictly religious people of his time obviously thought the health of the body was irrelevant in the general scheme of things. However he was not alone in this belief and he had some powerful historical figures on his side. For instance the medicine of the Tamil Siddhas, who did not view the body 'as a source of pain and temptation, but as the most reliable and effective instrument of man in his quest to conquer death and bondage. Since liberation can be gained even in this life, the body must be preserved as long as possible, and in perfect condition, as an aid to meditation, leading to freedom.'[4]

Buddhism can also be seen to share some of the Ayurvedic physician's respect for the body although perhaps for different reasons. Buddhists were keen students of medicine and their lack of taboos concerning the body made them particularly good at surgery.

From this we can see how Ayurveda medicine might come to play an important role in many areas of Indian culture, which was, at the time Caraka wrote, in a state of flux. In order to understand all this we need a summary of the medical doctrine as described in the lengthy - and not always easy to understand - medical treatises.

---

3   The *Caraka Samhitâ of Agnivesha* text and English translation by R K Sharma and B Dash (Chowkhamba 1988). I. 1, 6-17. hereafter referred to simply as CS.
4   K V Zvelebil, *The Poets of the Powers*, (London: Rider 1973) page 31.

Ayurveda and the West

Western physicians have always kept one eye on their Hindu counterparts. In modern times several summaries of the Ayurvedic system were made. One of the earliest was written by the eminent Indologist and diplomat H.H.Wilson, a pioneer in this field. Unfortunately his work was marred by the chauvinism of the nineteenth century observer.[5] For example he says:

The successful cultivation of the healing art by European skill and learning has left us nothing to learn from the Hindus.[6]

If this were true, them why did he go to such trouble to research it in the first place? Wilson concentrated upon the surgical developments of ancient Indian medicine. Despite his dismissal of Hindu medicine, many Indian techniques were taken up by European surgeons with some success. It may surprise you to learn that several operations in modern plastic surgery were first described in Ayurvedic medical texts. One of these is indeed called the 'Indian technique' and is a procedure to replace an amputated nose with a skin graft taken from the patient's forehead.

Before Wilson's essay, Royle, a professor of pharmacology, published a study of Indian medicine but it attracted far less attention than the famous diplomat. Royle describes the *materia medica* of the Ayurvedic tradition, finding that the range of drugs, both mineral and vegetable, as utilised by the ancient doctors was very large indeed.

Some years after this, a much more complete study was written by Dr J.Jolly, a physician practicing in India, who seems surprised and

---

5 H H Wilson, 'On the Medical and Surgical Sciences of the Hindu's,' *Works* Vol. III (London 1864), pages 269-276; 380-393.

6 *op cit.*, page 269.

almost put out that Ayurvedic medicine was still thriving:

> ...Despite *the advances by European medicine through English colleges and hospitals.*[7]

Another Way of Seeing

There is nothing miraculous about Ayurveda or the fact that it has survived so long. The reason it has done so is due in part to the rational, practical basis of its techniques. Ayurveda undoubtedly has its limitations but we may still learn much from it. It would be wrong to cut ourselves off from its knowledge in the mistaken belief that only one medical system, the western one, possesses all the facts.

Its very existence is a challenge to our preconceptions. Only the bigoted 'know it all' will dismiss non-western science without a proper hearing. However things are changing, especially in the medical domain. Western medicine is increasingly the subject of criticism from its own patients and practitioners. Perhaps then, the time is right to introduce some extra data from an unusual source.

The Basis of Life

The following account is based upon two medical encyclopaedias that were compiled in the first few centuries of the present era. Although they are the work of several authors, they are commonly known as the Caraka Samhitâ (CS) and the Sushruta Samhitâ (SS). It is not always easy to find English equivalents for some Ayurvedic terms. I will do my best, but please bear in mind that some words such as 'soul' are only roughly equivalent to the Hindu 'âtman'.

The Ayurvedic medical system takes an organic view of the world.

---

[7]   J Jolly, *Medicine*, (Strasbourg 1901). pages 1.

Medicine of the Gods 13

The Ayurvedic picture of things is of a highly dynamic biosphere. The parts of this biosphere are interconnected. The parts of the biosphere are also modifications of various structures underlying the nature of things. These things are known by simple experience. This is most obvious when one looks at Ayurvedic description of the kinds of disease:

Atreya, the legendary founder of the Ayurvedic medical school says:

Disease may be the cause that produces...another disease. For instance: Haemorrhage originates from the heat of fever, fever from haemorrhage and consumption from them both, etc. [8]

What Ayurveda calls a disease is to our western minds, often merely the surface symptom. This may lead to a noticeable difference between the types of diseases described in Ayurvedic and other medical systems.

In Ayurvedic medicine the basic underlying essence of the body is called 'rasa'. Rasa is basically a liquid which is found in various forms and is often the connecting link between various points in the system. References to rasa go right back to the Vedas where it is used to denote the essence of the Soma plant[9]). Soma was often identified with the moon. Soma was also a shamanic drug, gathered by moonlight, and had a white sap the colour, so it is said, of semen. In the Indian tradition the moon is also the abode of the spirits of the dead awaiting their re-entry into the cycle of rebirth and death.

The liquid rasa is present in our bodies and in nature, it is everywhere. It flows through the biosphere in a cascade. According to Caraka:

---

7   J Jolly, *Medicine*, (Strasbourg 1901). page 1.
8   CS II.8,16-19. See also chapter four for some further examples of disease categories of Indian medicine.
9   Edwin Gerow, *Indian Poetics* (Wiesbaden, 1977) In RV i,105,2 = semen.

The water present in the atmosphere is from the Moon. [It] is by nature cold and light and tasteless.[10]

It rains down from the atmosphere and [once] fallen is permeated with the qualities of the five-elements: it [then] nourishes the solid bodies of mobile and vegetative creatures; augmenting the six tastes [rasas] in their bodies.[11]

We have to look in religious texts to find out how the liquid rasa is supposed to get to the moon in the first place. The Brihad-Āranyaka Upanishad says:

When a man dies: They carry him to [be offered in] fire. His fire itself becomes fire, fuel the fuel, smoke the smoke, flame the flame, coals the coals, sparks the sparks. In this fire the gods offer a person. Out of this offering the person, having the colour of light, arises. Those who know this as such and those who meditate with faith in the forest on the truth, pass into the light, from the light into the day, from the day into the half-month of the waxing moon, from the half-month of the waxing moon into the six months during which the sun travels northward, from these months into the world of the gods, from the world of the gods into the sun, from the sun into the lightning [fire]. Then a person consisting (born) of the mind goes to those regions of lightning and leads them to the worlds of Brahma. In those worlds of Brahma they live for long periods. Of those there is no return. But those who by sacrificial offerings, charity and austerity conquer the worlds, they pass into the smoke [of the

---

10 CS.I.26,39 The Sanskrit phrase 'avyaktarasa' I have translated as 'tasteless' although literally it means 'unmanifested taste'.
11 CS.I.26,39b.

cremation fire], from the smoke into the night, from the night into the half-month of the waning moon, from the half-month of the waning moon into the six months during which the sun travels southward, from these months into the world of the fathers, from the world of the fathers into the moon. Reaching the moon they become food. There the gods, as they say to King Soma, increase, decrease, even so feed upon them there. When that passes away from them, they pass forth into this space, from space into air, from air into rain, from rain into the earth. Reaching the earth they become food. Again, they are offered in the fire of man. Thence they are born in the fire of women with a view to going to other worlds. Thus do they rotate. But those who do not know these two ways, become insects, moths and whatever there is here that bites.'[12]

All the substances in the world are usually analysed on the basis of their taste. Taste is probably the most important analytical tool in Ayurveda. There are six basic tastes:

Sweet (svâdu)
Sour (amla)
Saline (lavana)
Pungent (katuka)

---

12 BAU.VI.2,14-16 Translated by S Radhakrishnan (London, Allen & Unwin: London 1953). There are similar passages in the *Chandogya Upanishad* V.3-V.10,10, the *Bhagavad-Gîtâ* i,23-26 and several sections of the Mokshadharma. Food and the food chain is an important analogy for samsâra or the wheel of rebirth and death. See S. P. Collins *Selfless Persons - Imagery & Thought in Theravada Buddhism* (CUP 1982) page 211.

Bitter (tikta)
Astringent (kashâya)

We are perhaps only used to four primary tastes: sweet, sour, salt, bitter or acid. Any finer distinction may be based on the sense of smell, although subjects who have temporarily lost their sense of smell usually retain the ability to appreciate a great many subtle tastes, such as meat juice, fish, cheese and oranges.[13] The pungent taste as mentioned in Ayurveda may require an element of smell for its perception, whilst the astringent taste probably relies on the ordinary sensations of the tongue and not the taste buds at all.

From the medical point of view there are several further properties of an object that are worthy of attention. In addition to an object's taste, it has a substantial quality (dravya), a potency or effect (vîrya) and a secondary or reactive taste (vipâka).

Although substance is fundamental, taste is the most important manner in which to classify or analyse matter.

The 'Five Elements' (pañcamahâbhûta)

Substances come in five basic varieties: Space, Air, Fire, Water and Earth. These terms are translations of the Sanskrit words: kha[14] (or âkâsha,) vâyu, agni, ap and kshiti[15] The five were probably first

---

13 H T Anderson, 'Problems of Taste Specificity' pages 71-82, in *Taste & Smell in Vertebrates*, edited by G E W Wolstenholme and J Knight (Ciba Foundation Symposia, Churchill: London 1970).

14 'Kha': cavity or aperture is an interesting synonym for 'âkâsha': elemental space. One of its earliest occurrences is in the *Atharva Veda* xiv.2,1 & 6. Another meaning corresponds the English term 'canal' which is almost

15 CS.IV.1,27.

described together in such texts as the *Mahabharata*:

Then the water sprang into existence like something darker within darkness. Then from the pressure of water arose wind. As an empty vessel without a hole appears first to be without any sound, but when filled with water, air appears and makes a great noise; even so when infinite space was filled with water, the wind arose with a great noise penetrating through the water. That wind thus generated by the ocean of water, still moveth, coming into (unobstructed) space, its motion never stopped. Then in consequence of the friction of wind and water, fire possessed of great might and blazing energy, sprang into existence with flames directed upwards. That fire dispelled the darkness that had covered space. Assisted by the wind, fire drew space and water together. Indeed combining with the wind, fire became solidified while falling from the sky, the liquid portion of fire solidifies again and became what is known as earth. The earth or land in which everything is born is the origin of all kinds of taste, of all kinds of scent, of all kinds of liquids, and of all kinds of animals.[16]

---

16 The *Mahâbhârata* trans. by K Gangopâdhyaya and others. (P C Roy, Calcutta 1961). Shantiparva (Mokshadharma) Chapter 183. (Cannot locate this in the *Mahâbhârata* critically Edited by V S Sukthanker, S K Belvalkar & P L Vaidya (Poona 1927); See also Chapter 194 (187 in Critical Edition), 247-8 and Anugîtâ 50. certainly a derivative. It differs subtly from âkâsha: open space. One might even say that 'kha' signifies a particular space, and âkâsha: universal space.

The five elements as a whole is not a concept found in the earlier Vedic texts, although one does find several correspondences mentioned between natural phenomena and the parts of the body. These correspondences are sometimes seen as the forerunner of the five element theory:

> *On dying the human body must dissolve himself in nature: that the eye goes to the sun, the soul to the wind, to the sky and to the Earth according to the order...*[17]

Caraka the physician echoes this when he writes that:

> *'Man is a microcosm of the world'.*[18]

and

> *'Earth is the substance of that Man, Water the moisture, Fire the heat, Wind the breath, Space the cavities, Brahma the inner Self'*[19].

The five elements 'theory' seems to have been developed at the same time as the Ayurvedic medical system was put together. It is not an

---

17 RV.X.16,3. As quoted by Jean Filliozat, *The Classical Doctrine of Indian Medicine - Its Origins and Greek Parallels*, English Translation by D R Chanana (Delhi: Munshiram Manoharlal 1964). page 63.
18 CS.IV.5, 3 (a).
19 CS.IV.5, 5a.

unreasonable conjecture to suggest that the medical schools played some part, arguably even a key one, in its creation.

Disease 'infects' this world of the five elements. Every part of the physical body is made from a mixture of the five elements, although one element may well predominate in particular organs. Thus earth is said to correspond with the sense of smell; water with the sense of taste; fire with vision; air with touch or the skin and space with the ears and the hearing sense. But diseases are also know to trouble the Mind. This is possible because mind is also thought to be a substance, albeit a special one. Mind is formed from three proto or subtle substances called the three Gunas.

The Gunas: Three Strands of the Mind

Underlying the five gross elements of which the world and our bodies are made, are three qualities or 'proto-substances' known in Sanskrit as the gunas. It is easy to confuse these with the three humours described below, but they are subtly different. In Sanskrit the three gunas are - Sattva, Rajas and Tamas. These are difficult terms to translate into English although we do have some comparable triads such as essence, energy and inertia. A Hindu gnostic[20] text defines them as:

Of the nature of pleasure, pain, and delusion;[21]

---

20 F Edgerton in 'The Meaning of Sâmkhya and Yoga', *American Journal of Philology* 45 (1924). 1-46 was the first to suggest gnosticism as a possible translation for Sâmkhya, otherwise more often called the school of enumeration or classifying.

21 *Sâmkhya Kârikâ of Ishvara Krishna* and the *Tattva-kaumudî* (Vâcaspati Mishra's Commentary) trans. by (G Jha Poona 1934) XII Hereafter referred to as SK (Jha).

The 'sattva' attribute is held to be buoyant and illuminating; the 'rajas' attribute exciting and mobile; and the 'tamas' attribute sluggish and enveloping.'[22].

The manifest world of the elements (mahâbhûta) is caused by the blending and modification of the three gunas, 'like water'.[23] *This last point refers to the way the taste of water is modified in the atmosphere.*[24] *It is this same theory of taste (rasa) that was discussed earlier.*

The three gunas are of particular importance in Ayurvedic psychology. As mentioned above, Mind is a specialized substance and as such is also composed of the three gunas. It is the relationship between these in the constitution of Mind that gives rise to healthy or pathological temperaments. Thus Caraka says:

Rajas and Tâmas are the pathogens of the Mind.[25]

which can be compared with Patañjali's *Yoga Sûtras*:[26]

Yoga is said to be the restraint of the mental states (citta)[27]

---

22 SK XIII (Jha).
23 SK XVI (Jha).
24 SK XVI (Jha).
25 CS.I.1,57b.
26 J H Woods *The Yoga System of Patañjali: with Veda VyâsaYogabhâshya* and Vâcaspâti Mishra's *Tattvavaishâradî* (Cambridge, Mass. 1927). Hereafter called YS, YB and TV respectively. Patañjali's *Yoga Sûtra*, with Veda Vyâsa *Yogabhâshya* and Vâcaspâti Mishra's *Tattvavaishâradî* edited by J Vidyasagara (Calcutta 1874).

The Tissues of the Body

The body is obviously a lot more complex than five elements and three gunas. We must then examine the basic tissues of the body. Unlike Mind, which is a finished product after its manifestation in the foetus, the five elements have a protean quality, combining with each other in various permutations. A useful metaphor for this is the mixing of colours. From a basic White, Black and Grey arise the three primary colours Red (Rajas), Yellow (Sattvas) and Blue (Tamas). The mixing together of these primary colours gives rise to secondary colours or formations. Seven different tissues are mentioned in Ayurvedic texts: Fluid (rasa); Blood; Flesh; Fat; Bone; Marrow and Semen. We can add to this the three humours Wind (vâta); Bile (pitta) and Phlegm (kapha). The physicians recognized one further concept that they termed *Ojas*. This may be translated as bodily vigour[28] or the mysterious life force itself. Finally the impure waste products of metabolism: sweat; hair; urine etc. The above list covers all of the essential building blocks that could be discerned by the ancient Hindu physicians in the structure of the human body. It may seem simple but what they did with this model is simply amazing. In the next chapter we will see how they are combined together into a complete human biology.

---

27 YS.I,2 yogas cittavrittinirodhah

28 According to Monier Williams, *Sanskrit-English Dictionary Ojas* come from the root *vaj* or *uj* and means bodily strength, vigour or energy. Vajra or wand comes from the same root as does one of the epithets of Shiva - the terrible one - *ugra*. Related to this are Zend word *avjanh*; Latin *vigere, augere, augur, augus-tus, auxilium*; Gothic, *aukan*; English *eke*.

2
Health and the Origin of Disease

In Caraka's medical textbook,[1] he draws all of his sources together in the form of a dialogue. In it several elders of the Ayurvedic tradition discuss the origin of humanity and its diseases. Several divergent views on the origin of disease are discussed: some suggest âtman ('self') is the cause, another that disease is a mental phenomena caused by Rajas and Tamas (two subtle strands of matter). Yet another contends that disease is hereditary or due to actions in past lives. Another opinion is that God or time itself as manifesting seasonal change is the cause of disease. Although all of these things and more are thought relevant, the grand patriarch Atreya refutes them and states what has since become the authoritative explanation of the advent of disease.

In Ayurveda the very same thing that determines the healthy development of an individual is also responsible for a creature's downfall:

---

1 CS.I.25.

> Whatsoever produces growth beneficial (sampad) to man, those very (things) wrongly disposed (vipad) may set in motion numerous diseases.[2]

This common cause is food, the basis of health and ill-health. The eating of wholesome food brings health, whilst ill-health results from wrong eating.[3] Malnutrition is here taken in its widest sense and includes consideration of the quality of the food eaten and the manner of cooking etc. Also to be considered are its inner qualities. In addition, a food that may be thought in all other ways good such as milk or rice, may be unwholesome in medical terms if taken at the wrong times, or in inappropriate quantities.

In the stomach the food is divided into two portions; a pure liquid food called 'rasa' and the indigestible part or waste 'kittâ'. The rasa undergoes a series of metabolic changes within different parts and tissues of the body. This process can be likened to a cascade, as it flows through the body undergoing several transmutations. At each step in the cascade a waste product is produced. The form of this waste product is determined by the point in the system at which this happens.

Some of the waste products of digestion are actually quite useful to the good running of the system. Most important are the three humours - Wind, Bile and Phlegm.

The Three Humour Theory

'Humour' is a translation of the Sanskrit word 'dosha'. This term derives from the root 'dush', 'to spoil'. Whatever its original meaning may have been, many present-day Ayurvedic practitioners see the doshas as three life-forces.

---

2 CS.I.25,29.
3 CS.I.25,31.

It is well known that European medicine before the rise of the current clinical model, was also based on the humours. In the old European system there were four humours: Blood, Phlegm, Black Bile and Yellow Bile. In Ayurvedic physical medicine the Humours are three - Wind (vâyu or vâta), Bile (pitta) and Phlegm (shlesman or kapha), although ancient surgeons such as Sushruta included blood as an auxiliary or lesser 'humour'.

The three humours can be seen as *specialized* forms of the elements, Earth, Water etc., although with a subtle difference. The heat of digestion is obviously not the same as physical fire although they are related in some subtle way. In fact Caraka [4] separates them and treats Bile and Fire as two different things when he describes some patients as 'consumed by Bile, alkalis *and* Fire'.

The humours are bodily tissues composed of an admixture of all five elements. When we talk of the Pitta, the 'Fiery' Humour we really mean that fire predominates in its composition. Just as pepper is said to have a preponderance of the element fire in its makeup but also contains earth, water etc.

One revealing way in which to view the functioning of the humours is to look at them as 'matter in its right or wrong place'.[5] According to this theory a substance only takes on bad properties when it is in the inappropriate place. Thus the greasy bodily fluid that sometimes becomes a troublesome mucus excretion, is an essential constituent of the body when acting as a bodily lubricant in the joints. However when present in excess quantities and/or in the wrong place, for instance in the eyes or nasal passages, this is called a disease.

This way of looking at things has a strong basis in material reality. There is of course another important way of looking at the cause of

---

4 CS.I.22,33
5 Mary Douglas *Purity & Danger - An Analysis of the Concept of Pollution and Taboo* (RKP 1966).

disease - in terms of external agents such as micro-organisms. Whilst Ayurveda does not deny the usefulness of this other approach, it nevertheless calls upon us to shift focus to our own internal mechanisms and how they allow certain diseases to manifest. Western medicine is also rediscovering the value of this approach, for example recent clinical studies have shown that a depressed person is more susceptible to virus infections.

Many Ayurvedic therapies actively play on the ambiguous nature of disease. Some commentators feel that it is the taboo nature of some medicines that make them effective. For example garlic or even blood in the form of raw meat, is so efficacious as a medicine because it is so forbidden. However it is worth remembering that Ayurvedic physicians were advised during their training to *disguise* the contents of so-called 'taboo' medicines from the patients who might otherwise be reluctant to take them. It is therefore unlikely that such medicines were prescribed merely for the reason that they were taboo.

The three humours have a function within the body as well as a potential morbidity. We see this most clearly if we look more closely at the way in which these humours are said to transmutate within the body. For example there are said to be five sub-varieties of Pitta/Bile which arise out of the metabolic cascade. The Pitta present in the stomach (Pâcaka) aids digestion. If it is deranged then it gives rise to headaches and other illnesses. Following digestion in the stomach the digested food (rasa) passes to the liver and spleen and is there re-metabolized. The Pitta generated here is called 'rañjaka' and is responsible for the blood's red colour. If a defect occurs at this point then jaundice may result. Next the blood flows to the heart and is again re-metabolized. Pitta here is called 'sâdhaka' or the 'holder together'.

In classical Ayurvedic physiology the heart is the seat of consciousness. Most of us probably regard the brain as the seat of consciousness. Ayurvedic physicians are trying to alert us to the fact that the brain is not the *only* seat of consciousness. The western model of the 'Self' occupying the head like some ghost in a machine is surely only partially true. It is valid to view consciousness as inhabiting the *whole* body and its organ the brain, the spinal cord and the whole nervous system. In this sense the body is permeated by consciousness. There are many ways in which we think with the body and phrases such as 'the heart remembers' have some profound truth to them. The 'sâdhaka' Pitta in the heart is said to give excellence of memory.

The Tantriks, who were a widespread mystical sect specializing in erotic and body magick, posited a specialized nervous system distributed along the axis of the spinal cord. Here, so they contend, are approximately six depressions or 'chakras', which seem to have a rough correspondence to what we call the endocrine and autonomic nervous system. The precursor of the Tantrik system of chakras can be seen in the original books on Yoga. In a chapter which enumerates the 'siddhis' or miraculous powers, one is advised to meditate upon the 'nâbhichakra' or navel chakra in order to obtain knowledge of the body's construction.[6] The Tantriks, whose ideas were drawn from medical sources, make it clear in their writings that they regarded the upper head as the seat of higher consciousness, although consciousness was not confined there.[7]

During the next stage of metabolism the Fire or Pitta is termed 'âlocaka' and is found in the eye. The final stage leads to 'bhrâjaka' Pitta and is responsible for the sheen in healthy skin. In the table at the end of this chapter is set out the entire matrix of the humours' functions and morbidity.

---

6   YS.III,29
7   S Dasgupta *History of Indian Philosophy* (CUP 1932) Vol II, page 257.

The Ecology of the Humours

The ratio between the three humours in the body is susceptible to seasonal and geographical variations. An individual who is becoming out of harmony with these cyclical fluctuations in space and time can be the decisive factor that turns a vital humour into a toxin. In this highly complex biosphere, every person will have a place where they are at their most healthy; usually where they were born or spent their early years. Lucky is the person who can stay there, but reality is often less convenient. Of course a person can adapt to a new environment given time, and corrective measures can help here. A significant part of this natural state or constitution (Prakriti) is passed on from parents. The determination of ideal constitution is an important part of therapy, and the physician may take some time asking extremely detailed and seemingly irrelevant questions about lifestyle and background. The function of the Ayurvedic physician is to determine precisely the optimal environment for each individual within the biosphere. The physician should also be able to devise a corrective regimen for a patient who is 'out-of-phase'.

A story from my own experience illustrates this point. Whilst researching this book in India, I became a bit run down. The Ayurvedic physician I was studying with noticed and advised a tonic. In my particular case he thought I needed something from my normal diet and suggested that I eat a little meat and drink some alcohol. I did indeed follow his advice, although I found that Textured Vegetable Protein (TVP) had enough of the qualities of real meat to do the trick.[8]

An important cycle which one needs to take account of is the pattern of seasons in the year. The traditional division of the year in India is into two halves - a waxing and a waning year. It contains a hot season and a cold rainy season. This pattern works very well in South Asia, where most of the traditional recipients of Ayurveda still reside. But as

---

8   TVP is made from Soya, a plant whose therapeutic benefits as part of diet are steadily being rediscovered in the west.

knowledge of the system spreads to countries outside of Asia, the original schema needs adjustment. Individual physicians should have their own way of coping with this. I suggest below a variant based on UK climatic conditions and derived from some of our own folklore.

In India the height of the cold season is January-March and it is then that the watery Phlegm abounds and, if left unchecked by either diet or other measures, will give rise to many of the Phlegm diseases, such as Catarrh or Bronchitis. May to July is the Hot season's peak, and Bile abounds along with the diseases Chickenpox and Measles. The entire cycle is neatly represented by the following diagram[9] based upon Caraka [10] and Vâgbhata [11].

---

9 Francis Zimmerman, *La Jungle et le Fumet des Viandes* (Gallimard le Seuil 1982) page 47.
10 CS. III. 9, 125.
11 VG 12, 24-25.

The Indian Seasons and the Cycle of Humours and Tastes

Period of maximum bitterness

                        Period of maximum oiliness

———Wind———

++++++++++++Phlegm+++++++++++++

************Bile************

Acid	Salty	Sweet	Bitter	Astrin-gent	Pungent
Rains[12]	Autumn	Winter	Cool Season	Spring	Summer
Jul-Sep	Sep-Nov	Nov-Jan	Jan-Mar	Mar-May	May-Jul

---

[12] Many aspects of the Ayurvedic system were described by Albiruni, the tenth century Arab traveller. The seasons are ruled as follows:

Rains	Autumn	Winter	Cool Season	Spring	Summer
Moon	Mercury	Jupiter	Saturn	Venus	Mars

See Albiruni's *India*, English Translation by Sachau, Ch. LXXX

The above diagram also shows the seasonal effects on the six basic tastes. In the Ayurvedic system there is clearly a dynamic relationship between the humours and the tastes. It is still relevant because nowadays many of our food stuffs come from all parts of the world. However I suppose if one wanted to adapt this to Europe or the Americas some variation would be necessary. The main change would probably be a juxtaposition of Phlegm and Bile in perhaps the following manner:

Possible European Cycle of Humours and Tastes
————Wind————————————

**********Bile*************

++++++++Phlegm+++++++++

Autumn	Winter	Spring	Summer
Sep/Oct/Nov	Dec/Jan/Feb	Mar/Apr/May	Jun/Jul/Aug

The Ayurvedic physician Caraka tells us that:

Bile, which is oily, hot, sharp, liquid, sour, fluid and pungent is soon overcome by medicines having opposite qualities.

Wind, which is rough, cool, light, subtle, mobile, non-slimy and coarse, is reconciled by medicines having opposite qualities.

Phlegm, which is heavy, cool, soft, oily, sweet, immobile and slimy is relieved by medicines of opposite quality.[13]

We can see from this that the effect of each of the humours is counteracted by foods with a particular taste. The basic pattern looks as follows:

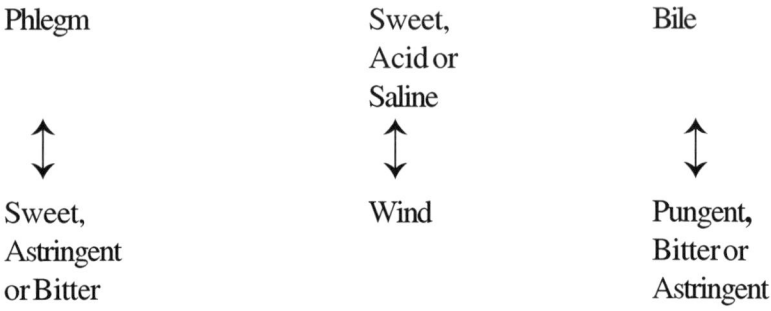

Key: -⁻ = tastes that are antagonistic to the given humours

This is a simple starting point. The basic polarity between the tastes and humours is a reflection of a botanical and biological frontier in India between the dry western territories of the Punjab - the 'Jangala' or dry soils. Opposed to these are the wet eastern territories, the 'anûpa' or 'swamp land'. Thus Consumption is a Bilious disease thought to be more

---

13 CS.I.1, 59-61.

common in the west. Fever, a Phlegmatic disease is more common in the east.

For general good health and mental equipoise any person is advised to take note of the relationship between the seasons and the characteristic of the food they eat in that season. For instance, during the winter months when Kapha is at its maximum, you should attempt to balance its effects with sweet, astringent or bitter foods. If you have manifested a disease of a serious type then a more complex therapy may be necessary and you need to consult a properly qualified physician. It is beyond the scope of the present work to advise on such cases. In general, the recommendation is to acclimatize a sick individual to the appropriate seasonal and geographical forces at work in any particular region. In any individual there will also be a particular equipoise of the humours that is natural for them, depending upon their constitution, age and lifestyle; this too must be taken into account in any therapy that aims to restore health. In addition the physician may apply one of the three special therapies designed to restore deranged humours:

There are traditionally said to be eight limbs of Ayurveda therapy viz.:

kâyacikitsa	Internal medicine
Shâlâkya	Treatment of head and neck
Shalya	Extraction of foreign bodies
Agadatantra	Toxicology
Kaumâra bhritya	Paediatrics
Rasâyana	Tonics
Vâjikarana	Aphrodisiacs

In addition three other important therapies are recognised, these are:

Sneha -   restoration of the vital oils of the body,

Sveda -   heat therapy involving application of

Samshodhana -   soothing poultices etc.

ridding the body's toxins by administration of purifying medicaments.[14]

The last of these can be quite extensive and includes the pañcakarma therapy or fivefold elimination of excess humours from the body.[15]

---

14 CS.I.14.
15 CS.I.2,15.

The Functions of the Three Humours

Vâta (located chiefly in the stomach region, see CS.I.20,8)					
Mode	Udâna	Prâna	Samâna	Apâna	Vyâna
Location	Throat	Heart	Stomach	Lower Body	Whole Body
Healthy function	Speech	Digestion	Digest-ion	Excretion	Aids liquid flow
Morbid function	Throat & heart disease	Asthma	Diarr-hoea	Diabetes	Fevers

Pitta (located in the intestines or âmâshaya)					
Mode	Pâcaka or Paktikrit	Rañjaka or Ragakrit	Sâdhaka	Âlocaka	Brâjaka
Location	Stomach and Intestines	Liver, spleen and stomach	Heart	Eyes	Skin
Healthy function	Digestion and secretion of rasa	Colours rasa to blood	Sight, determination and memory	Lubricates sense organs	Glazes and lubricates
Morbid function	Headache	Jaundice (kâmalâ)	Heart-burn	Conjunct-ivitis	Swellings

Kapha or Shleshman (located in the chest)					
Mode	Kledaka	Avalambaka	Rasana or Bodhaka	Snehana or Tarpaka	Shlesana
Location	Stomach	Heart	Tongue	Head	Joints
Healthy function	Moistens food	Firmness of limbs	Brings about taste	Lubricates sense organs	Lubricates
Morbid function	Loss of digestive power	Loss of appetite (tripti)	Goitre (galaganda)	Drowsiness	Stiffness

3
Temperament and Constitution

An animal is born with both a physical constitution (prakriti) and a mental temperament (sâra). Physical constitution is determined at conception by the predominance or otherwise of one of the three humours (dosha). These are Wind (vâta), Bile (Pitta) and Phlegm (kapha). The following summary is based upon Caraka's (Vimânasthâna). Immediately following the summary of the salient characteristics of each of the three basic types, I have appended the corresponding description as found in the work of the other great physician Sushruta.[1] The study of physical constitution was a crucial area of Ayurvedic practice and remains so in the present-day. Dr Ashvin Barot, an Ayurvedic physician practising in London, gave an almost word for word version of the classical account to the author.

---

1   English translation of the Caraka Samhitâ made by R K Sharma & B Dash (Chowkhamba Sanskrit Series 1976)   with some amendments of verses 95-99; The passages from SS.III.4,59-69; Bhishagratna translation.

The Unctuous or Watery Type
(shlesmala or kaphaja)

In key words Phlegm has the following qualities: It is
oily
smooth
soft
sweet
strong
thick
slow
stable
heavy
cold
slimy
clear

Each of these twelve properties imparts specific characteristics to the human body. The various parts of the body will be smooth, moist and well-formed. The complexion will be clear and the general appearance is very pleasing to the eye. Unctuous types have happy, outward-going personalities. The sweetness mentioned above will manifest itself in a man or woman as virility and a strong libido. The body will be very strong and compact with firm limbs and joints. Complementary to the body's strength is its plumpness. These individuals are slower than most others in several ways; appetite, physical reactions, temper and in movement.

Rather poetically, 'The complexion of the person of Unctuous temperament resembles either the colour of a blade of grass, blue lotus, a polished sword or that of the stem of the sara grass. He or she is comely in appearance, fond of sweet tastes, grateful, self-controlled, forbearing, unselfish and strong; he or she does not hastily form any opinion. and is fast in his emnity. The eyes are white; and the hair is curly and raven black. He or she is prosperous in life.

Their voice resembles the rumblings of a raincloud, or the roar of a lion or the sound of a drum. In dreams they often see large lakes or pools decked with myriads of full blown lotus flowers and geese. His or her eyes are slightly red towards the corners, the limbs are proportionate and symmetrical with a coolness radiating from them. He or she is possessed of all the 'sattva' qualities, capable of sustaining pain and fatigue and respectful towards his superiors. They possess faith in the scriptures and are unflinching and unchanging in friendship; suffering no vicissitudes of fortune, make large gifts after long deliberation, are true to their word and always obedient to preceptors. The traits of this character resemble those of Brahman, Tudra, Indra, Varuna, a lion, horse, elephant, cow, an eagle, goose and of the lower animals.'

The Fiery Type (pittala)

In key words the fiery humour is
hot
sharp
smells musty
or of raw meat
sour
pungent

It expresses itself in several physical characteristics and marks especially freckles, moles and port-wine stains. Such people will be physically strong and fleshy with a noticeably warm touch and natural tolerance of the cold. Their skin shows premature wrinkles and greyness. Before it becomes grey the hair is soft and brown, especially around the body. The libido is lower than in the previous instance along with fertility and fecundity. Due to the predominance of the Fiery humour digestion is strong and the appetite large. Unfortunately there is a tendency to develop unpleasant body odours and bad breath. People with this constitution can expect to thrive moderately well, with a reasonable length of life and material comforts.

'A person of the Fiery constitution perspires copiously emitting a fetid smell. Their limbs are loose, shapely and yellowish in colour. The finger nails, palate, tongue, lips, soles and palms of such a person are copper coloured. He looks ugly with wrinkles, baldness and grey hair; he eats a lot, is averse to warmth and irritable in temper, though he rapidly cools down again. He is a person of middling strength and lives up to middle age. On the plus side the person is intelligent and possesses a good memory and loves to monopolize the conversation. They are said to be vigorous and irresistible in battle. In dreams they see meteors, lightning flashes, fire, 'nâgeshvara', 'palâsha' and 'karnikâra' plants. They are fearless and do not bend before a powerful antagonist; They protect the supplicant and are very often afflicted with mouth ulcers. The traits of his character resemble those of a serpent, an owl, 'gandharva', 'yaksha', cat, monkey, tiger, bear and mongoose.'

The Air Type (vataja)
In key words Wind has the following qualities: It is
dry
light
mobile
abundant
swift
cold
hard
conspicuous

All this makes the bodily features, including the hair, nails, teeth and limbs, coarse in appearance. The joints are loose thus adding to the generally gangly look. The conspicuous quality manifests in the noisy action of the joints which creak and crack. The dryness can result in a stunted and emaciated body which is intolerant of the cold. Dwarfism also falls within the parameters of the pneumatic type. The voice is noticeably hoarse or even broken. This type of person will be light-footed and quick moving. Their reactions are very sharp. They are easily irritated and nervous. They grasp things fairly readily but often forget them. They are often quite talkative. The pneumatic type is the least desirable of the three and can expect the shortest life and few attainments.

'A [person] of the pneumatic constitution is wakeful, averse to bathing and cold to the touch. Unshapely, vain and dishonest. They are fond of music. The soles of the feet and palms of the hands are much fissured; A man may have a rough, grisly beard and moustache, finger nails and bodily hair. They can be hot tempered, prone to biting of finger nails and grinding the teeth. Impulsive, unsteady as a friend, ungrateful, lean and rough; the body shows a large number of surface veins. Sometimes incoherent and vacillating. A fast walker. In dreams they scale the skies. The eyes are always moving and the mind is never steady. They have few friends and are incapable of accumulating any money. The traits of this character resemble those of a goat, jackal, hare, mouse, camel, dog, vulture, crow or ass.'

All of these typologies reflect several traditional notions. For instance it can be seen that there is a significant polarity between the Unctuous type and the Pneumatic type. The paradigm is the unctuous type. In the Indian tradition to be 'stout' is a positive virtue and Bhîma, one of the heroes of the Mahâbhârata has the epithet 'vrikodara' or 'wolf-belly', because of the fact that his belly hung down. This 'stoutness' is carefully distinguished from obesity which is an unfavourable condition.[2] It is noticeable that today's Indian

---

2 CS.I.21,3.

filmstars, the modern-day role models, are much more rotund than their Hollywood counterparts.

Mental Temperament

In Ayurvedic psychology there are three basic personality types or temperaments. This classification is based on the three gunas or 'reals' that underlie any substance. For a more detailed exposition on this subject the reader is referred to Mitchell Wiess's study of 'Unmâda' or insanity.[3] There is very little difference between the accounts of Caraka and Sushruta on this score and I will be following Caraka's version.[4] He tells us that Mind comes in three varieties - Sattva, Rajasa and Tamasa.[5]

'The Sattva Mind is said to be free from defects, because of its extreme perfection. The Râjasa Mind is defective because of its extreme wrathfulness. The Tâmasa Mind is said [to be] defective because of its extreme ignorance.'[6]

The structure of Mind in Ayurvedic psychology is very similar to the tri-partite soul of Platonism (See *The Republic* IX.580e[7]). The Soul is said to possess reason, passion and appetite. In Caraka (as incidentally in Plato) the three basic types yield sixteen possible personalities dependent upon simple permutations of the basic three. Each of the sixteen is given the name either of a spirit (bhûta), a sacred individual or of an animal. This provides us with an

---

3 M Weiss, 'A Critical Study of Unmâda in Early Sanskrit Medical Literature.' (University of Penn, Thesis 1977).
4 CS.IV.5,36-40. SS.III,4,74-76.
5 See YS.II.18.
6 CS.IV.4,36 For parallel passage see SS.III.4,74-75.
7 Plato: *The Republic* English translation by Paul Storey (London, 1961).

interesting clue to the manner in which the Ayurvedic physicians sometimes viewed the categories of spirits drawn from the manifold archetypes of Indian culture, as fairly precise personality types. Rather like the present day psychological terms such as 'Oedipus Complex', 'Uranian Syndrome' and 'Hermaphrodite'.[8] In the table on page fourty-one I have set out the three basic orders of the personality and underneath each have put the sub-varieties. The reader will instantly recognize the affinity between this basic threefold classification of personality and the same distinction widely drawn in Tantrik texts.[9] The suggested English equivalents to the Sanskrit archetypes, are partly derived from the work of Mitchell Weiss[10] with some additions of my own. Caraka never intended this list to be exhaustive and he in fact comments that the number of actual personality types is extremely prolific. For those interested, it is possible to make correspondences between the following typology and the lunar parts of Indian astrology.[11]

---

8 First Suggested by Bhagavat Sing Jee *A Short History of Aryan Medical Science* (London 1896) page 202.
9 Arthur Avalon (Sir John Woodroffe) *The Serpent Power* (Dover 1974) page 53. The threefold Tantric classification of personality is into Gods (divya), Heroes (vîra) and Beasts (pashu). This can be compared with the theories of W H Sheldon, *The Varieties of Human Physique* with S S Stevens & W B Tucker (New York 1940).
10 *op cit* page 95.
11 M Magee, *Tantrik Astrology: A Manual of Sidereal Astrology*, (Mandrake, Oxford 1989), page 12 and page 83-87.

The Personality Types of Ayurveda

Sattva Mind	Rajas Mind	Tamas Mind
Brahma (godly)	Asura (demonic)	Pashva (bestial)
Rishi (sagely)	Rakshasa (aggressive)	Matsya (fishy)
Indra (authoritative)	Pishaca (Manic depressive)	Vanaspatya (vegetative)
Yama (restained)	Sarpa (retilian/deceitfull)	
Varuna (courageous)	Preta (morbid)	
Kuvera (generous)	Shakuni (officious)	
Gandharva (ecstatic)		

Some of these personality types are associated with the lunar parts of Indian astrology. The Brahma type with the day of the full-moon; the Rshi and Asura with dusk and dawn; the Râkshasa with the moon's dark fortnight and the Preta with its bright fortnight. [12]

---

12 M Weiss, *op cit* page 198.

4
Common diseases of Ayurvedic medicine and their ancient antecedents

The aim of this chapter is to *contrast* earlier Vedic ideas on disease and healing with the Ayurvedic theory of disease causation and classification of diseases. This is only possible if one first isolates a purely Vedic doctrine of medicine, something that is not readily available from the work of most Vedic scholars, whose primary concern was to trace later doctrines back to their supposed genesis. Kenneth Zysk's recent study of Vedic medicine does not adopt the usual viewpoint where 'in almost every work, Vedic medicine was evaluated in terms of the later tradition of Ayurvedic medicine'.[1] The

---

1 Kenneth Zysk, 'Early Vedic Ideas of Disease and Healing with translations and Annotations of Medical Hymns from the *Rig Veda* and *Atharva Veda*' (Ph.D. Australian National University 1981).

Ayurvedic system, which dates from about the sixth century before the common era until the present day, should be clearly distinguished from the Vedic system that it superseded. There are significant contrasts between the two medical systems and these suggest to me a number of intriguing hypotheses. One possible explanation of any change in the type and frequency of disease may be changes in ancient society itself. That is to say, changes in disease somehow mirror social changes in ancient Indian society. The mechanism of change is well known and has been described in many important books, including those discussed below. If we for a moment see things from the 'disease's' point of view, one has an organic entity with a particular environment which is most favourable to its survival. Some diseases, such as Malaria or Tuberculosis, are endemic in specific geographic or demographic situations. Changes in the environment, whether natural or man-made will favour some diseases and hinder others, perhaps changing the situation sufficiently so that a disease that was at one time epidemic becomes endemic.

The Ayurvedic medical system supersedes the large mass of medical ideas exhibited in the Vedic texts. The differences in perception of disease between the two systems (if it is permissible to call the Vedic one a system) are evidence not merely of a philosophical change, but of a change in material conditions, making certain diseases or frequencies of disease possible. The two main material changes that are relevant to this study are: firstly, the movement of peoples, as in the case of war and

---

'Religious Healing in the Veda', *Transactions of the American Philosophical Society* Vol. 75 part 7, 1985.

2   W. McNeil, *Plagues & Peoples* (Blackwell 1977).
    H. Zinsser, *Rats Lice & History* (Bantam 1965).

expansion; and secondly, the urbanization of and growth of centres of population. The effect of both these phenomena have been studied in several general works of medical history and social history of disease. The two classic works are William McNeil *Plagues and Peoples*, and H Zinsser's earlier *Rats, Lice and History*.[2] Both these works inspired me in the attempt to make some similar speculations concerning the dialectic of disease and social change in ancient India.

The ancient Vedic view of disease was essentially rural or pagan.[3] Vedic categories of disease are much broader, as well as fewer in number. Diseases, when manifest, were usually self limiting or amenable to fairly simple remedies; either that or their resolution was rapid. Zysk says that 'the ancient Indian concept of internal disease was based upon the fundamental notion that illnesses were caused by demonic entities which entered the body. Each demon had a specific name and caused particular morbid bodily conditions.'[4] For example 'Yákshma', one of the commonest disease categories of Vedic times, is related to Yaksha, a supernatural being.[5] All this is in marked contrast to the Ayurvedic doctrine, where classes of disease are extensive and the causes of disease, with some notable exceptions, are almost wholly naturalistic, that is to say they were not connected with demonic possession. The only exceptions to this are the incurable aspects of any particular disease as well as some diseases of childhood, with the possible addition of some mental disorders.

---

3 Latin: 'Paganus' = country dweller.
4 Zysk. *op.cit.* page 8.
5 A Coomaraswami, *Yaksha* (Washington: 1928).

Diseases of the Vedic 'system'

On the basis of the *Bhaishajya* section of the Kaushika Sûtra, Zysk has reconstructed a basic classification of ancient Vedic diseases. He finds that Vedic diseases fall into three main groups:

i) Internal diseases related to Yákshma and/or Takmán, i.e. wasting and febrile conditions.

ii) Internal disease not closely related to Yákshma/Takmán, e.g. worms.

iii) External diseases, e.g. fractures.

I. The Yákshma/Takmán Complex of Diseases

1. Yákshma

This is a disease that afflicts both humans and cattle with a generalized wasting of the body. Most authorities concur in the identification of this disease as some form of Tuberculosis, or to give it its more archaic name, Consumption. Indeed, Caraka himself recognizes this fact and includes the Vedic disease Râjayakshmâ as a subspecies of Shosha. The more precise clinical notes found in Caraka Samhitâ[6] enable a conclusive translation of these terms to be made. The *Atharva Veda* records an incantation to *magically* counteract the effects of this disease. It would

---

6 CS.II.6,12.

be wrong to suppose that Vedic therapy was restricted to purely sympathetic magic. In *Atharva Veda* 19.44 1-2 an ointment (áñjana) is recommended for various diseases including Jâyânya and Yákshma. The Sanskrit 'añjana' is a collyrium, either antimony trisulphide or lead sulphide. Compounds with a great number of medical applications are found within the later Ayurvedic period.[7]

> *[1] From your eyes, from (your) nostrils, from (your) ears, from (your) chin, from (your) brain, from (your) tongue, I tear away from you the yákshma which is in the head.*
>
> *[2] From your neck, from (your) nape of the neck, from (your) vertebrae, from (your) spine, from (your) shoulders, from (your) forearms, I tear away from you the yákshma which is in the arm.*
>
> *[3] From your heart, from (your) lungs, from (your) hálikshna, from (your) two sides, from (your) two mâtasnas, from (your) spleen, from (your) liver, I tear away from you the yákshma*
>
> *[4] From your bowels, from (your) intestines, from (your) rectum, from (your) stomach, from (your) pelvic regions, from (your) plâshì. from (your) navel, I tear away for you the yákshma*
>
> *[5] From your thighs, from (your) knees, from (your) heels, from (your) forefoot, from (your) haunches, from (your) bhámsas, I tear away for you the yákshma which is in the backside.*

---

[7] *Mâdhanavadâna and its chief commentary*, with introduction, translation and notes by G Meulenbeld (Leiden 1974) page 438.

[6] From your bones, from (your) marrows, from (your) tendons, from (your) blood vessels, from (your) hands, from (your) fingers, from (your) nails, I tear away for you the yákshma.

[7] By means of Kâshyapa's exorcising spell, I tear completely away the yáksma which is in your skin, which is in your every limb, every hair (and) every joint.

The above is a very catholic description of the disease. It is in fact true that Tuberculosis can 'invade almost any organ, being seldom found, however, in the muscles or in tissues with few blood vessels, like *cartilage and sinews.*' I doubt if it is really possible to make the specific identification of Pulmonary Tuberculosis on the basis of verses from the *Atharva Veda*, although evidence of skeletal and visceral Tuberculosis is found in human remains dating back to 4000BCE.[8] As an instance the verses cited by Zysk are as follows:

'*Be not afraid; thou shalt not die; I make thee one who reaches old age; I have exorcised the yákshma, the waster of limbs, from thy limbs, the splitter of limbs, the waster of limbs, and the heartache that is thine, the yákshmâ hath flown forth like a falcon, forced very far away by (my) voice*'[9]

'*Limb splitting, limb-wasting and vishalpaka of all the limbs every head-disease etc.*

---

8   R Y Keeb, *Pulmonary Tuberculosis A Journey Down the Centuries* (Tindall, 1978).
9   *Atharva Veda*, translated D Witney (Harvard Oriental Series, 1905) 5.30 8,9.

Of whom the fearful aspect makes a man tremble the takmán of every autumn we expel out (of thee) by incantation.

The yákshma that creeps along the thighs, that goes also to the groins, from thy limbs within we expel etc.[10]

It seems only valid to say that yâksma was a very general category of wasting disease that perhaps included some of the more severe manifestations of conditions now classified along with Tuberculosis. The significance of this fine distinction will become more apparent when we examine the progress of the disease in Ayurvedic times.

2. Jâyânya

This is a disease demon particularly associated with yâkshma. There is no agreement among scholars as to the type of disease meant. K Zysk says that 'it was a type of yákshmâ which enters the body and by the fact that it causes the belly to enlarge, it may be a kind of congenital disease, the most common being 'congenital heart disease' or a type of disease suffered particularly by women.'[11]

3. Kshetriyá

An 'exact' description of this disease is not given in any of the charms. Again, there is no general agreement among commentators as to a possible translation. Indian authorities consider it to be some sort of intractable hereditary disease.

---

10 AVS 9.8.5.
11 Zysk *op cit.* page 20.

4. Rápas (Disease)

A general internal disease-entity, the equivalent of the later Sanskrit *roga* (disease). Zysk's analysis of its occurrence in the Vedic texts shows that it is often used in connection with diseases and deformities of the feet.

5. Hriddyotá, Harimán

'Heart-pain' and 'jaundice' The strange juxtaposition of these two diseases or symptoms in the texts indicates that at least in some cases the yellowness is associated with the heart-pain or *vice versa*. On the level of sympathetic association we can say that heartburn and yellowness are both 'fiery' type phenomena. Both disease entities are also encountered separately.

6. Balâsa (swellings)

A symptomatic swelling commonly associated with internal diseases. Again this is a very broad definition and most examples of secondary swellings come under this category, including swelling of lymph nodes and possibly herpes or fever sores.

7. Takmán

Zysk confidently translates tâkman as malaria and in this he is in step with most other commentators. The principal symptoms are fever and coughing, which are manifested in the rainy season. As Zysk himself comments, coughing is not one of the notable symptoms of malaria except in 'the advanced stages of the most severe types of the disease.'[12] The ascription of such a precise definition may be slightly

---

12 *op cit.* page 74.

misleading and the more cautious will be happy to give it the broad definition of fever, with the possible inclusion of malarial fever. An interesting point is that the principal cure is the kushtha plant. in Ayurvedic times this venerable herb also gives its name to a whole class of skin disorders including leprosy,. Unless there is a complete change of meaning, this implies that the Vedic therapy was often aimed at the symptoms, which were 'fever sores' or herpes simplex.

8. Kasa

Cough, closely associated with takmán. In addition to the eight disease categories above there are a number of general charms concerned with several secondary symptoms of the above yákshmâ/takmán complex. These include such things as ear-ache, stomach-ache and skin disorders.

II Other Internal Diseases

1. Amîvâ

This is a very general disease entity that gives rise to bodily wasting and malnutrition, and in certain circumstances, abortion.[13]

2. Víshkandha-Sámskandha

There is no clear translation for this disease entity. Zysk is the first to suggest that it might refer to Tetanus, although this is debatable. Tetanus was one of the diseases mentioned by the Greek philosopher Plato in his supposed early account of the Ayurvedic medical system.[14]

---

13 RV 10.162.
14 Plato *Timaeus* 84d-86a (see page 86 above).

3. Udára (Dropsy)

In the Vedic Samhitâs there are no specific hymns or charms which themselves are devoted to the cure of dropsy, which only in the later medical literature is included under the general category involving a swelling of the abdomen called *udara*. The most we have are scattered references to an abnormal bodily condition which seems to suggest dropsy.[15]

4. Únmadita and únmatta

This is insanity[16] There were two main causes of this condition; in the case of únmadita the mind-loss is due to infringement of rules or taboo. In later cases, demonic possession is the cause.

5. Krími:[17] (Worms)

The word 'Krími' does not occur in the *Rig Veda*, although the *Caraka Samhitâ* shows the continued interest in the study of worm related diseases, the only common term is for *dantâda*[18] worms, or worms in the teeth. A universally common inference perhaps drawn from the shape of the decayed cavity. The records of the Buddhist physician Jîvaka[19] bear a close relationship to the Vedic practice in this matter. One text describes a treatment of head-disease by trepanning the skull and removing a troublesome worm.[20]

---

15 RV 7.89, AVS 1.10.
16 AVS 6.111.
17 AVS 2.31 & 5.23.
18 From Skr *Dat*, hence Latin *Dens* etc.
19 See C Morgan, *Buddhism and Ayurveda*, (forthcoming).
20 *Mahâvagga of Vinaya Pitaka*, chapter 8.

6. (Urine retention)
The description of this condition and its remedy is found in AVS 1.3.

III External Diseases
These are less clearly defined and the charms are not all devoted to human medicine. Some of them are obviously meant for the treatment of animals.

1. (Fractures)
cf: AVS 4,12

2. Haemorrhage, especially menorrhagia[21]

Let those young women, the hirâ (blood) vessels, clothed in red garments, who proceed as brotherless sisters, stop with their beauty drained.

> Stop, you lower one; stop, you upper one and also stop, you middle one. And (since) the smallest one stops, indeed the dhamáni (blood) vessel should (also) stop.

> Of the hundred dhamáni (blood) vessels (and) of the thousand hirâ (blood) vessels, these middle ones have indeed stopped. Jointly, the end ones have come to rest.

> The solid bank of sand,[22] has surrounded you (O vessels); stop,

---

21 AVS 1.17.

remain perfectly still.[23]

3. Skin disorders

i. Pálita, Kilâsa, i.e. leukoderma, white patches on the skin, the result of various skin disease.

ii. *Apacíts* is a pustulating rash, probably the same as found in Sushruta.

iii. Hair-loss, especially in women.

If a comparison is made between the main disease categories of the Vedic Samhitâs, as reconstructed by Kenneth Zysk, and the main categories as found in the Ayurvedic Samhitâs of Caraka and Sushruta, some interesting features emerge from the comparison. Zysk feels that the external diseases of Vedic medicine were more obviously based on physical experience. On the whole the Vedic categories of disease are far less well defined than those found in the later Ayurvedic texts. Many of the translations have to be taken as provisional. It is difficult to form any picture of the prevalence of any particular disease in Vedic times. Zysk himself feels that an individual disease-entity may get a mention as much for its severity as for its incidence.[24] However, a careful comparison between the Vedic and Ayurvedic lists reveals the manifestations of what may be some new diseases. The following diseases are either not mentioned in the Vedic Samhitâs, or if they are it is by a different name and/or under a much less specific category:

---

22 Perhaps a reference to the application of a poultice of warm sand.
23 Zysk, *op cit.*, page 225.
24 Private Communication.

The New Diseases of Ayurvedic Times

1. Consumption (It is debatable whether the Vedic disease-entity Yákshma is identical to the Ayurvedic Shosha.)
2. Tumours and cysts
3. Diabetes
4. Leprosy
5. Epilepsy
6. Nervous diseases
7. Piles
8. Urinary calculi
9. Fistulas

This is not a comprehensive list, but it covers several of the more important disease categories identified by Caraka and Sushruta in their respective diagnostic textbooks (Nidânasthânas). It is of course possible that the perception and attention to disease may also have altered. However there is no reason to maintain that this could be or was the only reason for the differences between Vedic and Ayurvedic medical experience.

Ayurvedic diseases and their possible social significance

1. Shosha (Consumption)

Tuberculosis, the modern equivalent of Consumption, is still, and perhaps always will be, the scourge of the planet, with millions of deaths each year. Modern drugs have given us in the West perhaps only a temporary respite from the disease. Most scholars agree that the real inroads against the disease came before the discovery of the modern antidote, and were brought about by public health measures. However in one state of India alone (Uttar Pradesh) 513,007 cases were treated in one year and there were 642 mortalities.[25] The World Health Organization estimates that there are as many as twenty million cases, which annually infect 50-100 million people.[26]

The disease is described in the sixth chapter of the Nidânasthâna of the Caraka Samhitâ. According to Caraka there are eleven symptoms of Consumption: heaviness of head (shirasah paripûrnâtvam), coughing (kâsa), indigestion (shvâsa), hoarseness of voice (svarabheda), vomiting of phlegm (shleshmanashcchardanam), spitting of blood (shonitashtîvanam), pain in sides of chest (pârshvasamrojanam), grinding pain in the shoulder (amsâvamarda); fever (jvara); diarrhoea (atîsâra), and loss of appetite (arocaka).[27]

These symptoms are comparable to what modern clinical medicine calls pulmonary tuberculosis, which in the early stage gives rise to coughing, spitting of blood, sweating, sickness, diarrhoea and constipation. In later stages the spit is thick and yellow and the victim becomes greatly emaciated. Vomiting and diarrhoea become more frequent. Caraka records four main causes of the above condition:

1. Overstraining (sâhasa)
2. Suppression of natural urges (samdhâranam), e.g.

---

25 *Government of India Statistical Abstract, 1978*: 'Diseases Treated in Hospitals and Dispensaries for 1970'. Those familiar with the Ayurvedic medical geography might like to compare this with West Bengal where 40,538 patients were treated and there were 344 mortalities. The population of Uttar Pradesh was then 88.25 million, and of West Bengal, 44.25 million.
26 H T Mahler, *Tuberculosis in the World Today*. (Bull. Int. Union Tuberc. 43.19. 1970).
27 CS.II.6,14.

eructation
3. Wasting (kshaya)[28]
4. Irregular diet (vishamâshanam)

From our point of view the last of the above causes is the most interesting:

When a man consumes drinks, foods and lickables neglecting wholesomeness, dietary rules, time, quantity, geography, combination, preparation and nature, then because of this their Wind, Bile and Phlegm becomes imbalanced. These then spread all over the body, obstructing the mouths of the channels of circulation, so that whatever food is taken by that individual is mostly converted into faeces and urine rather than bodily tissues. The afflicted man therefore becomes constipated.

Wind *produces colic, malaise, irritation of the throat, pain in the sides of the chest, grinding pain in the shoulders, hoarseness of the voice and head colds.*

Bile *causes fever, diarrhoea and burning sensations inside the body.*

Phlegm *causes head colds, heaviness of the head, loss of appetite and coughing.*

Due to excessive coughing there is injury to the chest and the

---

[28] From root kshi, 'to wane', as applied to the moon. This particular disease is said to afflict men who are too attached to their sexual partners, or whose love is unrequited. The condition is related to supposed pathological semen loss.

patient spits blood. Because of the discharge of blood he becomes weak.

Thus the three humours accumulated due to irregular dieting manifest the disease Rȃjayakshma.[29]

In this final sentence Caraka identifies Ayurvedic 'Shosha' with the Vedic disease-entity 'Yȃkshma' described earlier. The symptoms given in the Vedic medical hymns are much more vague and general than those given in Caraka's description. This leads me to speculate that Caraka is drawing the parallel on the basis of the severity and prevalence of consumption in his time. Although Shosha was not precisely the same disease as Yȃkshma, it was to Caraka equal in severity, thus he called it a Rȃjayȃkshma or *King of diseases.*[30]

Experts in western clinical medicine regard Consumption or Tuberculosis as essentially a social disease. According to the *Textbook of Medicine*, 'a situation favourable to acquisition of infection would be an overcrowded and poorly ventilated house.'[31] It is a disease 'commoner among the ill-fed and the badly housed. In Britain the abolition of overcrowding, provision of good homes, an adequate supply of protective foods and enough money to buy them have gone a long way towards diminishing the incidence of Tuberculosis.'[32]

The presentation of this disease in Ayurvedic texts provides a clue to

---

29 CS.II.6,10.
30 'Captain of All the Men of Death' John Bunyan quoted in R & J Dubos *The White Plague*, (Gollancz, 1953).
31 *The Cecil Textbook of Medicine*, 17th edition by J Wyngaarden & L H Smith (London 1985) page 1621 (hereafter referred to as Textbook of Medicine).
32 'The Epidemiology of Tuberculosis' in *Tuberculosis*, G P Youmors (Saunders, 1979).

understanding the social environment in ancient India. For all the facts show that whilst Consumption is one of those diseases that can persist in small isolated communities, it can become epidemic when urbanization occurs and large numbers of susceptible people become involved. 'Many conditions are known to increase the risk for the recurrence of tuberculosis. Among these are emotional stress, malnutrition, influenza, pneumonia and cancer of the lung.'[33] All of these factors are noted by Caraka in his etiology of the disease. One could also note the fact that it is now known that Bovine Tuberculosis is able to infect humans via unpasteurized milk.

2. Diabetes (Prameha)

The fourth chapter of Caraka's *Nidânasthâna* is devoted to the analysis of diseases that manifest themselves as abnormalities in the urine. Analysis of urine is one of the most important diagnostic tools of Ayurveda, as it is in most other medical systems. Variations in its amount, colour, odour, specific gravity, reactivity and deposits are revelatory of several different conditions. Caraka lists twenty different disorders of the urine, grouped according to the humour that is chiefly involved.

1. *Phlegm*
    i) udakameha (watery urine)
    ii) ikshuvâlikârasameha
        (sugarcane urine: temporary Glycosuria)
    iii) sândrameha (thick urine)
    iv) sândraprasâdameha (Urine with thick residue)
    v) shuklameha (white urine)

---

33 *Textbook of Medicine* page 1622.

    vi) shukrameha (white deposits)
    vii) shîtameha (cold urine)
    viii) sikatâmeha (stones)
    ix) shanairmeha (urine retention)
    x) âlâlameha (slimy urine) [34]

2. *Bile*
    i) kshârameha (alkaline urine)
    ii) kâlameha (black urine)
    iii) nîlameha (blue urine)
    iv) lohitameha (red urine)
    v) mañjishtameha (light red/smoky tinted urine)
    vi) haridrâmeha (yellow urine) [35]

3. *Wind*
    i) vasâmeha (fat urine) [36]
    ii) majjâmeha (marrow urine) [37]
    iii) hastimeha (copious urine) [38]
    iv) madhumeha (sweet urine) [39]

The diseases revealed in this list of twenty conditions of the urine, have many equivalents in the western clinical model. This does not mean we can safely ignore those phenomena that aren't recognised by western clinical medicine. The whole purpose of studying alternative medical systems such as Ayurveda, is precisely because they contain hidden or

---

34 CS.II.4,10.
35 CS.II.4,25.
36 CS.II.4,41.
37 CS.II.4,42.
38 CS.II.4,43.
39 CS.II.4,44.

lost knowledge about our bodies and the world we inhabit. These systems have some extremely refined observations that we would do well to rediscover for ourselves. For example the study of dreams and other early signs as a method for the early diagnosis of disease is highly developed in Ayurveda. These kind of symptom are not unknown even within western clinical medicine, which calls them prodromal symptoms. However their use could be extended.[40]

Urinary disorders arising from vâta (wind) are said by Caraka to be the most serious and virtually incurable. The early description by Indian physicians of the disease now called Diabetes (madhumeha) is a fact acknowledged by all modern histories of the disease. Diabetes Mellitus is not one disease but a heterogeneous disorder with multiple causative factors. Diabetes Insipitus is a pituitary disorder and therefore is a distinct disease entity. The complex of symptoms arising from deranged wind (vâta) is clearly a form of Diabetes.

In *Nidânasthâna* IV, Caraka enumerates an extensive list of actions that aggravate the humoural wind, displacing it from its proper function and giving rise to the four stated symptoms. The list includes bad diet and regimen.

> *'The aggravated wind in the affected body spreads along with the fat, when it enters the channels (that) carry urine, Oily-urine (vasâmeha) then arises. When so much of this has accumulated in the bladder (mûtrâshaya), marrow urine (majjâmeha) results. When there is excessive lymph and tossing about of deranged Wind, a constant desire for urination, the urine trickles away slowly like an intoxicated elephant. This is known as Elephant-urine (hastimeha). If at any time the Wind because of its*

---

40 See Chapter five

roughness assails with astringency the Ojas,[41] *which is naturally of a sweet taste, it carries it to the bladder and then causes 'sweet-urine' (madhumeha).*[42]

Modern Data on Diabetes

The following information from western clinical medicine is included here as it provides some interesting points of comparison. According to modern wisdom, Diabetes Mellitus is 'the commonest endocrine disorder. Prevalence in urban societies is 2-6%, many people being unaware of their condition. The disease is commoner in prosperous societies and among certain races.' It is now widely believed that many groups of Indians are predisposed to Diabetes, given a suitable environment.[43]

Cause

1. Genetic endowment is important in those contracting diabetes. In all age groups environmental factors may determine which of the genetically pre-disposed develop clinical diabetes.
2. Age: 80% of cases occur in those over 50 years.
3. Obesity and diabetes are associated but uncertainty exists as to whether obesity causes or results from diabetes.
4. Physical stress may induce diabetes in susceptible people.

Clinical Features

Diabetes affects the metabolism of proteins, fats, carbohydrates, water

---

41 See comments on *Ojas* in chapter one. If we accept that *Ojas* is the conceptualization of the body's vital energy, then the allusion here may be to potential fatalness of *madhumeha*.
42 CS.II.4,37.
43 *Diabetes in Epidemiological Perspective*, Mann, Pyorala & Teuscher (Churchill Livingstone. 1983) page 47.

and electrolytes. Without the secretion of a sufficient amount of insulin, glucose cannot pass into tissue cells and instead accumulates in the circulation with the following results:

1. The blood glucose level rises (hyperglycaemia).

2. The kidneys are unable to reabsorb all the glucose passing through them and glucose appears in the urine (glycosuria).

3. The high concentration of glucose in the filtrate exerts an increased osmotic pressure which hampers the reabsorption of water by the renal tubules, so that a much larger volume of urine than normal is formed (polyuria).

4. Polyuria leads to dehydration and thirst. The patient drinks large quantities (polydipsia).

5. Fat is utilized for energy production instead of carbohydrate, but is incompletely metabolized since for its total combustion, carbohydrate must be metabolized simultaneously. Toxic acid products of incomplete fat metabolism (ketones) accumulate in blood and urine and are also excreted in breath, giving it a characteristic smell.[44]

3. Tumours & Cysts

The third chapter of the *Nidânasthâna* is devoted to the description of a broad category of tumours and cysts. The Sanskrit word for this special type of swelling is *gulma*, which as a medical term is uncommon in texts prior to the Mahâbhârata.[45] There are said to be five varieties of gulma, four of which arise from complications of deranged humours. The fifth arises from blood and is a gynaecological disorder.

Hippocrates used the term *karkinos,* to describe a similar group of diseases characterized by uncontrollable cell growth or development.

---

44 *Understanding Nursing Care*: ed. Anne M Chilman & Margaret Thomas; p 385 (2nd ed. Churchill Livingstone, 1982).

45 M Monier-Williams *A Sanskrit English Dictionary* 1st Edition (Oxford 1899) 'gulma'.

As in the Hippocratic tradition, gulmas can be divided into the categories of benign or malignant. The causes of gulma are mainly complications of wind for such as bad food or physical trauma of several kinds, e.g. suppression of natural urges, physical assault, constipation or lack of exercise. *Sâmnipâtika gulma*, i.e. that which arises from the vitiation of all three humours together, is a very severe and incurable condition. Ayurvedic *gulma* and modern cancer are probably the same disease. Western clinical medicine has no commonly agreed explanation as to its cause although certain varieties of cancer are statistically more common amongst certain sexes and dispositions, occupations, social classes, in specific localities and in those exposed to certain traumatic events. Ayurvedic gulma has many points of similarity with some of the modern cancers of the lower bowel and organs. There are thought to be dietary factors involved in its inception, perhaps also lack of dietary fibre.[46]

4. Leprosy (Hansen's Disease)

The fifth chapter of Caraka's *Nidânasthâna* describes a broad category of diseases under the eponym *kushtha*, which includes leprosy. There are two main groups of factors in the genesis of leprosy: (i) disorders in the three humours (Wind. Bile and Phlegm) and (ii) disorders in the tissues (skin, muscle, blood and lymph. The Ayurvedic description again coincides with the current division of leprosy into Tuberculoid leprosy and Lepromatous leprosy. The former is usually confined to a small area of the skin and its nerves, and the later involves a massive infection of the dermis.[47]

---

46 *Textbook of Medicine* page 1072.
47 *Textbook of Medicine* page 1634.

Medicine of the Gods 67

Complications arising from the three humours include the often observed numbness particularly associated with humoural 'Wind', which is the functional equivalent of what we term the nervous system. Before the use of sulphones in 1941, the main treatment for leprosy was chaulmoogra oil (hydnocarpus oil) a therapy plainly derived from Ayurveda. *Black's Medical Dictionary* records an ancient Burmese folk story that 'a Burmese prince who discovered chaulmoogra oil in the treatment of leprosy'.[48] A more reliable if less picturesque source than Black's, says that the western name comes from a very rare Greek word meaning a nourishing fruit. The fixed oil is expressed from fresh ripe seeds of Hydnocarpus wightiana, H. anthelmintica [presumably meaning used to treat worm infestations], and also Taraktogenos kurzii. This latter species is named after the Sanskrit name for the oil, *Tuvaraka*.[49] It was most commonly administered by direct infiltration of the lesions, and thus encouraged resolution, It may have prevented some indeterminate and early borderline forms of leprosy from progressing into the lepromatous type.[50] According to modern clinical medicine there is no evidence to show that Leprosy is due to any dietary deficiencies. However according to Caraka, these are the main causes of the condition.[51] Leprosy is very slow to develop and is only very slightly contagious. A necessary condition for any significant manifestation of the disease would be a population of sufficient density to engender frequent contacts with contagious pus in its 'open' phase. Leprosy is not known in the *Atharva Veda*. Its true history begins in the later population centres of the Indus in the early post-Vedic period.

---

48 *Black's Medical Dictionary*, 35th ed. 'Leprosy' (hereafter called *Medical Dictionary*.
49 SS.Cik. 13,20.
50 Abstracted from *Martindale's Extra Pharmacopoeia* 28th edition by J. E. F. Reynolds and A B Prasad (Pharmaceutical Press: London 1983) pp. 1492-3.

5. Epilepsy

Epilepsy (apasmâra) is one of the diseases noted in the Nidânasthâna and the condition was well known in all ancient cultures where records have survived. In modern times it is estimated that about one person in twenty has a fit of some sort in the course of a lifetime, but only one in eight who have a fit will suffer from chronic epilepsy. The causes of the condition are obscure; there is a certain degree of family incidence of the disease, although only about 4% of children of affected parents develop the condition. 'Among precipitating factors which are influential in the development of epilepsy in predisposed individuals may be sudden fright, prolonged mental anxiety, overwork and alcoholism'[52]

6. Piles

The celebrated Ayurvedic surgeon Sushruta described one or two diseases that were largely ignored in the work of Caraka, who was not a surgeon.[53] Nevertheless the underlying causes of these conditions is metabolic, and several of them reveal some quite interesting features of the ancient Indian lifestyle. Today it is estimated that by age 50, 50% of people will have them.[54] Piles (arshas) are described in the second chapter of Sushruta's *Nidânasthâna*. There are said to be six main classes: those arising from disorders of one of the three humours, either

---

51 CS.II.5,6
52 *Medical Dictionary*: 'Epilepsy.'
53 See C Morgan, *Buddhism and Ayurveda* (forthcoming) for an examination of the differences between the Ayurvedic surgical and physical traditions.
54 *Textbook of Medicine* page 785.

singly or all together; those due to blood disorders, and those of a congenital nature. The term 'Piles' is normally restricted in clinical medicine to the varicose and inflamed condition of the veins at the lower end of the bowel. Sushruta's classification of arshas extends to warts as found on the genitals of both sexes, as well as other parts of the body including the eyelids. It is common nowadays to divide piles into three varieties: internal, or those afflicting the mucus band just inside the anal sphincter; external piles occur under the skin just outside the bowel, and mixed Piles occur on the sharp line between the skin and the mucus membrane of the lower bowel. In the main, habitual constipation is the principal cause of piles and this is the chief cause identified by Sushruta in his pathological comments. The first line therapy for Piles is the addition of bran to the diet.[55] This is not actually mentioned by Sushruta as a cure, although in the recommended convalescent diet, no meat is included as it is in other conditions. In the Caraka's *Cikitsâsthâna* VI,7 the diet is to be wheat barley, Shashtika rice or Shâli rice, etc.

7. Renal Calculus

Stones (ashmari) are described in some detail by Sushruta in the seventh chapter of his Cikitsâsthana. There are three types of bladder stone, according to which Humour is involved. Alleviation was sought by the use of various decoctions in order to dissolve the stones *in situ*. 'Stones originating in the bladder are rare in industrialized countries, although they were common in antiquity and are still frequent in certain countries in South East Asia.'[56] Not surprisingly Sushruta says that the most common variety of calculi occur in the bladder, and if the above remedy

---

55 H Thomson, 'Piles: Their Nature and Management.' *Lancet* 2:494 1975.
56 *Textbook of Medicine* page 620.

fails, surgery is advised as a last resort. So precarious is the surgical procedure that the permission of the king was required, as death under the knife was to be expected.[57] In common with the ancient physicians, modern wisdom also recognizes three types of calculus: *Uratic* is associated with acidity or with the gouty constitution. Although the causes of this acidity are unknown, it shows a marked hereditary factor. It is also widely believed that it is more common amongst those of sedentary habits, which apparently gives a greater opportunity for the stones to crystallize. Some other precipitating factors are undoubtedly inadequate exercise, luxurious manner of living, habitual overindulgence in animal food, rich dishes and especially in alcoholic drinks.[58] Excessive intake of calcium, i.e. dairy products is also a factor in the inception of this disease.

The second type of bladder stones are *Oxalic*, composed of oxalate of lime, and often associated with a nervous dyspeptic type of temperament. And thirdly, *Phosphatic*, which occur in long-standing cases of inflammation of the bladder. This is now the most common type of stone found in the bladder.

Conclusion

With one or two arguable exceptions, the diseases of the Ayurvedic period differ markedly from those presented in the earlier Vedic period. I have not attempted to analyze every one of these new diseases, but some of the main categories, in order to facilitate the formation of a general view. Several passages show that Caraka the physician viewed the emergence of these diseases as a catastrophic event. For instance, in the *Nidânasthâna* he renders the Puranic myth of the destruction of

---

57 SS.Cik 7,30.
58 *Medical Dictionary* 'Gout'.

the Daksha's sacrifice. In this widespread motif, the god Shiva (Maheshvara) in revenge for not being invited to Daksha's sacrifice, sacrifices Daksha! Sometimes it is said that Shiva was angry because Daksha or Brahma's feast was an incestuous wedding sacrifice. In the ensuing chaos the following diseases were engendered: gulma (tumours), prameha (diabetes), kushtha (leprosy), unmâda (insanity), apasmâra (epilepsy), raktapitta (haemorrhage) and râjayakshma (consumption).[59] The destruction of the Daksha's sacrifice is one of the quintessential myths of the Epic period of ancient Indian history.[60] In my opinion the myth is an attempt to explain the fact that all these new diseases have appeared. Ayurvedic medicine is one response to these new diseases. And it is Indra, a god with many affinities with Shiva, from whom the patriachs first obtained the means to combat those diseases.

The key point I wanted to make in this chapter is that these new diseases are social diseases and they arise in the well-known social changes of the five or six centuries before the beginning of the Christian era. The incidence of Pulmonary Consumption and Leprosy points to population density, especially in large urban centres. Arguably Cancer, Insanity and other nervous diseases are also products of the pressures of urban life. If there is an 'Indian disease' it was and still is Diabetes. We have seen that diet and lifestyle are of particular importance in the genesis of this condition; especially bad diet, including overeating. Diet also plays a part in two common, if less serious diseases of the times: Piles and Calculi. Perhaps they point to a surplus of food production or increase in the quantity of food available. The widespread consumption of dairy and meat products was not something new to this period, but there may well have been differences in quantity rather that the variety

---

59 CS.II.8,11.
60 Wendy O'Flaherty, *Asceticism & Eroticism in the Mythology of Shiva* (OUP, 1973).

of the food eaten. There is some indication of lack of fibre in the diet.

The Ayurvedic response to this new matrix of causes and disease has a much wider significance. Any medical viewpoint is inextricably bound up with what we can broadly characterize as a philosophical position. It is of course not the case that the Ayurvedic stance was the only one adopted in response to changing circumstances. Buddhism and other reform movements can make similar claims. However, the influence that Ayurvedic ideas exert on the new ideology constructed at this time is very significant, and will be discussed in a future volume in this series.

5
Food

Sushruta's catalogue of meats

The theory of Ayurvedic states that all food articles may be divided into two broad categories, determined by the climatic features of the animal or vegetable's habitat. The two categories are called in Sanskrit Jângala and ânûpa. The term Jângala is the Sanskrit cognate of the English term 'jungle' however, the commonplace conception of 'jungle' is the exact reverse of Sanskrit meaning, where it signifies the 'dry soil' terrain, flat with thorn bushes and the occasional tree. The counterpoint to Jângala is ânûpa or 'swampland'. In ancient Egypt a similar distinction applied to the futile 'blackland' and the relatively infertile 'yellow land'. In the Indian subcontinent these two regions roughly correspond to the western and eastern sections; that is to say there is a reasonably clear climatic polarity between the western and eastern tracts of the subcontinent. The east receives a much heavier monsoon than the west. This polarity is bound to be traceable at all levels of plant and animal life; as any gardener will know, some plants thrive in wet conditions whilst others perish. We can reasonably expect that this would affect the environment of micro-organisms and thus would correspond to a phyto-geographic gradient. The best example being the fact that malaria is epidemic in the west and endemic in the east.

An added complication to this is that the 'sanskritisation' or 'aryanisation' of the subcontinent progressed from the North-western parts towards the East and South. The war-like âryans took possession of what were for them the premium territories, which were originally 'Jângala'. Thus the battlefields of the Mahâbhârata are called 'kurujângala'. The expansion of the iron-age through the Indian sub-continent, through the process of conquest and migration, had the natural tendency of reifying the polarity 'Jângala' and 'ânûpa' into mental categories sometimes divorced from geographic facts. Francis Zimmerman shows in his book that the two usages overlap to a significant extent. Thus the divisions of the plant and animal kingdom on these lines does at least begin on a rational basis.

The catalogues of Caraka and Sushruta are catalogues of meats (mâmsa-vargah). Strictly speaking, what we are dealing with is more culinary in construction than zoological. Nevertheless this text can be compared to Aristotle's De Partibus Animalium[1] ('On the parts of animals'). The system of classification devised by Aristotle lasted for 1,400 years, after which it was gradually superseded by more empirical schemas. Aristotle based his classification on a type of comparative anatomy, ignoring the surface features, which he thought mere accidents, in favour of comparison of the supposed essential features of an organism. Thus instead of classifying animals on the basis of whether or not they have wings, he groups them into those with and those without blood. Birds, amphibians, reptiles and fishes form one genus; cephalopods, crustaceans, insects and testaceans another. These can be further classified by genus and species. His method led him to an awareness that whales, dolphins and porpoises did not belong amongst the fish category. The disadvantage of Aristotle's system is in the fact that it ignores surface details and is really only a lexical classification. Zoological and botanical definition was revolutionized by Carolus Linnaeus (1707-1778).[2] He made use of the hitherto neglected small parts of the flower, the features thought merely accidental by the Aristotelians. By shifting the gaze to the surface features of an object, he laid the basis for the empirical classification of plants and animals. His system was more practical as he successfully devised workable keys, making it possible to identify plants and animals from a book.

Aristotle is said to be the founder of scientific classification. However, the Ayurvedic system does have certain advantages over the Aristotelian one. As mentioned above, the two basic categories are determined by the climatic conditions of the animal's habitat - Jângala or ânûpa. Subsequent classification is into eight basic behavioural categories. Aristotle would have regarded an animal's behaviour as purely accidental. However, a classification based on these surface features is in modern eyes perfectly sound and close to the spirit of Linnaeus.

In Sushruta these are viewed as eight divisions of the basic Jângala genus. Separately from this he gives the ânûpa category six further subcategories. The most seminal version of the classificatory schema is that of Caraka, which has fewer inconsistencies.

Sushruta's eight divisions of Jângala animals are:
1. Those which have legs   (janghâla)
2. Those which scatter   (viskira)
3. Those which peck   (pratuda)
4. Those which have a lair   (guhâshaya)
5. Those which tear food   (prasaha)
6. Those which dwell in trees   (parnamriga)
7. Burrowing animals   (bileshaya)

8. Domestic animals　　　　　　　　　(grâmya)

His six categories of ânûpa animals are:

1. Animals that dwell on river banks (kûlucara)
2. Floating animals (plava)
3. Crustacea (koshastha)
4. Animals with feet (pâdin)
5. Fresh water fish (nâdeya matsya)
6. Marine fish (sâmudrâ matsya)

Although Sushruta's classification enumerates a few extra varieties of creature, it suffers from several ambiguities. For example, lions and tigers are not included amongst the category of animals that snatch their food (prasaha) - which includes other carnivores - for the reason that they are included in a separate category of animals with a lair (guhâshaya). [see appendix for full list of animals].

Caraka's catalogue of meats

A similar catalogue presented in Caraka's compendium is more succinct and does not suffer from the ambiguities of Sushruta's list; Caraka sticks to eight basic categories. They are:

1. Animals that snatch their food　(prasaha)
2. Burrowing animals　(bhûshaya)
3. Animals of marshy lands　(ânûpa)
4. Aquatic animals　(jalaja)
5. Floating birds　(jalecara)
6. Animals of dry lands　(Jângala)
7. Scatterers or Gallinaceous birds　(vishkira)

8. Birds that peck   (pratuda)[3]

The gallinaceous (vishkira) category of birds is further divisible into two sets - lavas etc and vartakas The distinction between these two types of bird lies in their respective habitats. Quail are from the dry lands (Jângala) and are thought to be the best gastronomically. Vartakas are bustards and live in wetter terrains (ânûpa), and have a heavier quality.

The translation of the catalogues of Caraka and Sushruta as given in the appendix is only provisional. There is especial difficulty in getting agreement on the lists of birds, whose species are extremely numerous, far more than are recorded by Caraka and Sushruta. The two lists of birds do not coincide completely. In the main, I have recorded the translations as given by R K Sharma and Vaidya Dash in their translation of the Caraka Samhitâ. I have amended this in some instances with some of the interpretations in Francis Zimmerman's catalogue drawn from Sushruta.

There is also the problem of the sheer number of animals that present themselves for classification. A good example of the problems of translation is the term 'sharabha', which is found in the Sushruta catalogue amongst the first group of animals, those with long legs (janghâla) and in Caraka with the animals of the dry terrain (jângala). In the Kâlikâ Purâna, the sharabha is the name given to one of the aspects of the god Shiva. He is said to be 'a terrifying beast with eight legs, some on top and some on the bottom'[4]. It seems unlikely that either Caraka or Sushruta thought they were classifying such a creature when they drew up their lists of deer. Sharma and Dash translate 'sharabha' as 'wapiti': Cervus Canadensis, but as Francis Zimmerman points out, this particular species of deer has never been an inhabitant of South Asia. For the time being it is best left as an unidentified variety of large deer.

On the sources of these catalogues we can only speculate.

Unlike Aristotle, there is no record of either Caraka or Sushruta actually engaging in the systematic study of zoology, notebook in hand. However as was noted on above, Aristotle also occasionally documents what appear to be mythological animals such as the 'Indian Dog'. Even if both catalogues are purely academic constructions, this would tend to limit their usefulness rather than completely empty them of zoological value. As with the entire compendium, they would be sensible redactions from several sources such as previous lists, dictionaries, names in other texts and the editor's own experience. Many of the names given to animals are onomatopoetic as in ulûka: owl or behavioural as in dindimânavaka: barbet; and this itself is evidence of some degree of observation. It is important to note that although both Caraka and Sushruta enumerate about two hundred animals, they only record the medicinal properties of a small percentage. The text demonstrates a respectable interplay between a formal system of classification and the way it impinges on experience. There is an extensive list drawn probably from several sources. A list which enables one to place any particular creature and predict its therapeutic properties. Drawn from this is a short resumé of meats that have been found actually of value in a therapeutic situation. Elsewhere Caraka gives a list of the animals that need to be to hand in a well-equipped clinic. They are:

quail	(lâva)
partridge	(kapiñjala)
rabbit	(shasha)
black buck	(harina)
antelope	(ena)
black-tailed deer	(kâlapucchaka)
red deer	(mrigamâtrikâ)
wild sheep	(urabhra)

milch-cow   (gâm dogdhrîm)[5]

The above list of animals also shows that Caraka did follow his own theoretical precepts. All of the above animals are from selective categories; group one (animals that snatch), group six (animals of dry terrain) and the first subsection of Gallinaceous birds (lavas, etc). Apart from the milch cow, all of the edible animals are drawn from classes thought by Ayurvedic theorists to have similar therapeutic properties. The meat is light, cold in potency, sweet with an astringent after-taste. They are useful antidotes to deranged humours, especially Bile .

Francis Zimmerman, to whose work I have already made several references, says that Sushruta's catalogue of meats, and by implication Caraka's, is not a zoological or scientific document; it is closer in character to a bestiary. A bestiary is a piece of medieval scholasticism, a treatise on beasts possessed of a highly moral tone. The purpose of these texts was not to teach anything concerning the animal kingdom, but rather to use the characteristics of certain beasts to illustrate moral points. The zoological content of these texts is purely incidental and thus in most instances entirely spurious. A bestiary abounds in completely mythological beasts such as the unicorn. There are several examples of medieval bestiary in the British Library. In one of these there is a picture of the mythical Caladrius, a bird that was said to alight on a sick person's bed. Symbolically the bird is often seen as a harbinger of death and if the Caladrius looked away from the patient then he would almost certainly die.[6] The Caladrius is a purely literary conceit; its presence on the margin of a fictional romance gave the reader a sign of the story's eventual outcome. This comparison arises from a suspicion that the Ayurvedic texts harbours mythological beasts. If this were true then the rationality of the catalogue would be in question and one would be left with a catalogue of purely literary, moral or cultural qualities.

One mythological suspect was already mentioned - the sharabha. There are, according to Zimmerman, several others, for instance the timi, timingila and makara. These three animals are included amongst the classification of marine fish (sâmudra matsyâh). These are all varieties of sea-monster, the 'makara' sometimes described as a beast with jaws of crocodile and body of a fish. However, given the already stated difficulty in re-identifying some of the species mentioned in the catalogue, I think one must give these creatures the benefit of the doubt. The deep oceans still to this day contain 'mysteries', and more so in the time of Caraka and Sushruta. It seems reasonable to give these terms the provisional translation of whales, dolphins or crocodiles; after all, the biblical term 'leviathan' is still used by Europeans as an synonym for the whale.

Even supposing that there are one or two mythological beasts in these catalogues, most of them are made up of recognizable natural species. The length of these lists is hardly exhaustive although they do list most of the available options. The basis of these lists seems quite rational. It would only be damning if Caraka or Sushruta went on to recommend the meat of one of the mythological beasts as a therapy - something never done in India, although there are some examples in the European tradition.

Caraka's catalogue of cereals

Caraka's classification of the staple ingredients of ancient Indian diet is also of interest. Cereals (shûkadhânya) are divided into six groups:

1. shâli   (winter rice)
2. shashtika   (60 day rice - summer rice)

3. vrîhi   (autumn rice)
4. shyâmâka (millet)
5. yava   (barley)
6. godhûma   (wheat)[7]

Shâli rice comes in many varieties. According to Cakrapânidatta's commentary on this section, Shâli rices are suitable for growing in the winter season (hemanta) which covers the two months of November and January. Referring to the diagram in chapter two, it will be noted that this is the time of the year when the sweet taste (rasa) predominates in the biosphere and consequently the three humours are in a state of equipoise. Thus shâli rices are said to be cold in potency and sweet in taste. They do not aggravate any of the humours and they are generally beneficial to the organism. Thus this season and the cereals grown during it are highly prized.

The second group of rice-cereals are Shashtikas. According to Cakrapânidatta, they are suitable for growing in the hot summer season (grîsma) which falls in May and June, just before the rains (varsha). The rice takes its name from the sixty-day growing period.[8] This is another point at which the three humours are relatively low and the crops take on the qualities of the season: they have a cold potency, are oily, light and sweet; and like the season, generally beneficial to the body.

The third group of rice-cereals are vrîhis. According to Cakrapânidatta, they are suitable for the autumn growing season (sharad) which is September to November, just before the premium winter months. Bile (pitta) is prevalent during this season although Wind and Phlegm are relatively low. So although it has a sweet taste in the mouth, its taste after digestion is sour and it becomes heavy on the system. Rice crops grown during this season aggravate the humours, especially Bile.

The fourth group, millet, etc (shyâmâka) are astringent and

sweet in taste; light, they counteract Bile and Phlegm but provoke Wind.

The fifth group, barley (yâva) have a rough as opposed to oily quality. It is cold, non-heavy, sweet and astringent. It provokes a great deal of Wind and counteracts Phlegm.

The sixth group, wheats (godhûma) are oily and cold with a sweet taste. They destroy Wind.

The above classification is based upon several formal notions developed within the Ayurvedic tradition. The first of these is the seasonal cycle of humours and tastes as described in chapter two above. According to this system the year is divided into six seasons. Each season is thought to be dominated by a particular taste (rasa). These, in turn, through their affinities and aversions, give rise to an ebb and flow in the amount of humours present in the biosphere and its organisms. Thus winter (hemanta), when sweetness abounds, is the time when humoural Bile is at its lowest level. We noted above that shâli rice was harvested in this season and consequently takes on its qualities. It is very sweet and good for the body. The idea that a food article takes on the medicinal properties of its environment is an idea largely ignored in the West. As stated it appears to be a purely formal notion with no basis in own modern experience. However the Ayurvedic theorists use these catagories in such a way as to suggest that experience did play some part in the construction of the model. There are *ad hoc* amendations of the formal rules, amendments that appear to have been dictated by practical considerations. For instance according to the rules of the system, any sweet taste will unfavourably increase the amount of Phlegm in the organism. Thus following the ultra-sweet winter season, Phlegm begins to increase. In typical manner Caraka tells us that there are a number of exceptions to this rule. At the beginning of chapter 27 of the Sûtrasthâna he says:

'As a rule sweet (things) aggravate Phlegm, with the exception of honey, and old shâli and shashtika rice, barley and wheat.'[9]

This is one amongst many such demonstrations of the way the Ayurvedic theorists used their theories and allowed them to be moderated by experience. Common sense tells us that living organisms do take on some of the qualities of the environment in which they live, especially through their food. For example the wide difference in taste between free range and battery-produced hen's eggs; perhaps ancient people were more sensitive to these kinds of environmental influences.

Differences in the order and length of the catalogue of cereals indicate the preference for some crops over others. There is possible indication here of the well-known juxtaposition between rice and wheat. In the East, where there is a greater abundance of water, rice growing predominates. In the north-west and south, which are much drier, the staples are crops such as wheat, barley and millet. Given Caraka and Sushruta's origins in the north-west of India, one would expect them to show a prejudice in favour of their local crops - wheat, millet and barley. If anything there is a bias in favour of rice as a staple food. This comes as no surprise considering the widespread delectation of this crop throughout Asia. What may be noteworthy is the fact that both Caraka and Sushruta were based in the northwest of India where rice would have been an eastern import. This shows some degree of objectivity applied when constructing this catalogue of cereals. If they had adhered to purely formal geographical criteria they would have ranked wheat as the premium food crop, but if anything, the opposite is the case.

Rationality and ayurvedic medicine

Jean Filliozat, characterized Ayurveda as 'a dogma which interprets experience.'[10] Abstractions, formal systems, matrices and tables abound in Ayurvedic texts. In F Zimmerman's more recent study, the author attempts to strip bare the essential formula lying at its heart. Following in the footsteps of Filliozat, he contends that Ayurveda is a variety of Rationalism, almost, to use his term, a 'clerical science'.[11] In the history of Western philosophy `Rationalism' is reserved for the seventeenth century metaphysicians - Descartes, Spinoza and Leibniz. They took as their starting point human reason alone, holding that 'the general nature of the world could be established by wholly non-empirical demonstrative reasoning.' In seventeenth century Europe, such a view was a breath of fresh air in the scholastic seminary, where divine reason and authority was the sole guide to the nature of reality. However, in the years that followed, pure reason was rejected in favour of the twin poles of knowledge: reason and experience.

Thus in our day Rationalism is pejorative. Francis Zimmerman tells us that in Indian medicine 'all the concrete information, all the empirical data, pharmaceutical, physiological and nosological are rigorously subordinated to the play of language.'[12] The 'play of language' in this instance signifies the play of a formal system. The subordination of empirical data etc by language is the function of a good theory; with the proviso that the theory should not smother the evidence. A theory may be thought objectionable when it degenerates into a mere play on words.

Judgments of the kind made above are controversial. 'The problem of the culture boundedness of meaning; of the universality of the criteria of rationality as it has developed in Western society; of the comprehensibility of ritual acts - have come into the full focus of a many-sided debate conducted between philosophers, sociologists and anthropologists.'[13] A tentative conclusion of this debate is that the categories of other cultures are not always translatable into our own, although they do often appear to be

Medicine of the Gods 85

derived from a more limited range of experience and from less comparative opportunity.[14] The aim of this chapter is to test out some of these assumptions by examining some of the catagories of Ayurveda. How far do they form a rational system and is the range of experience more limited than some of those categories in our own medical systems?

For Zimmerman the fundamentals of Ayurveda are encapsulated in its catalogue of foodstuffs. In Ayurveda, what one eats is the basis of health or the absence of 'Whatsoever (when) wholesome may cause the growth of creatures, when that is unwholesome may set in motion various diseases in man.'[15]

In both Caraka and Sushruta whole chapters are dedicated to the description and classification of food items, vegetables, meats and accessories.[16] The bulk of Zimmerman's study is devoted to the catalogue of meats as presented by Sushruta. Sushruta's catalogue is slightly longer than Caraka's, it includes one hundred and sixty-eight animals, ten more than in the Caraka version. It is also more complicated than Caraka's in its basic categories.

The formal analysis of taste

It should be clear by now that the relationship between the tastes is of great importance in the Ayurvedic medical system. Our primary experience of the food we eat is its taste and, closely related to this, its smell. As was pointed out earlier, the nexus of health or the absence of it lies in the food we consume;[17] Ayurvedic medicine has no real theory of infection as we know it. The food that we eat is digested in the stomach and reduced to one of three products: liquid food (rasa), waste (kitta) and the three humours - Wind (vata), Bile (pitta) and phlegm (kapha). When these humours are in their proper measure and place they are essential constituents of the body. For instance, the Bile facilitates the process of digestion rather like what we would call an enzyme. However, when any of these three humours becomes deranged it constitutes the underlying cause of disease. The question I intend to address is, what constitutes a state of derangement? Is it purely a theoretical notion or does it have some empirical content? In the Sûtrasthâna, Caraka goes into some detail on this score. He describes sixty-two permutations of the three humours that can be described as derangement and which therefore lead on to the manifestation of clinical symptoms. In what is a prime example of terse 'sûtra style', the brief verse acting as hardly more than an aide-mémoire. It was the duty of the physician to be able to recite the list in its entirety:

> *'There are six situations in which one finds either one or two humours excessively deranged. There are six situations in which one finds one or other of the humours slightly deranged, with another moderately affected and another very deranged. There is only one situation in which all three humours are deranged to the same degree'*[18]

The thirteen situations have then to be constructed from memory.

Diseases where either one or two humours are excessively deranged
1. Wind and Bile excessively deranged, Phlegm slightly deranged.
2. Bile and Phlegm excessively deranged, Wind slightly deranged.
3. Phlegm and Hind excessively deranged, Bile slightly deranged.
4. Wind excessively deranged, Bile and Phlegm slightly deranged.
5. Bile excessively deranged, mind and Phlegm slightly deranged.
6. Phlegm excessively deranged, Wind and Bile slightly deranged.

Diseases where the humours have a gradient

7. Wind slightly deranged, Bile moderately deranged, Phlegm most deranged.
8. Wind slightly deranged, Phlegm moderately deranged, Bile most deranged.
9. Bile slightly deranged, Phlegm moderately deranged, Wind most deranged.
10. Bile slightly deranged, Hind moderately deranged, Phlegm most deranged.
11. Phlegm slightly deranged, Kind moderately deranged, Bile most deranged.
12. Phlegm slightly deranged, Bile moderately deranged, Wind most deranged.

Diseases where the humours are deranged to the same
13. Wind, Bile and Phlegm excessively deranged.

This list does not appear to demonstrate any empirical knowledge, merely a recitation of thirteen logical permutations that any schoolchild could produce given simple instructions. The list appears to be purely a formal one of permutations and a demonstration of the supposed Indian predilection for list construction. Note here should be made that along with the celebrated medical texts of the Bower manuscript were found two short manuals on cubomancy and the arrangements of four and sixfold permutations. If we symbolize the above it may help us to see the logical pattern that lies behind the list. Let 'A' represent the humour in its 'slightly deranged' situation (hina). Let 'B' represent the humour in its 'moderately deranged' situation (madhya). Let 'C' represent the humour in its 'excessively deranged' state (adhika). Thus any of the three humours can be in state 'A', 'B' or 'C'. The entire matrix is as follows:

Wind   (vata)   A B C
Bile   (pitta)   A B C
Phlegm (kapha)   A B C

Permutation number one in the above list - 'Wind and Bile excessively deranged and Phlegm slightly deranged' would be symbolized as C C A. The thirteen permutations when written symbolically look like this:

C A C C A A A A C B B C C
C C A A C A B C A A C B C
A C C A A C C B B C A A C

A close inspection of this list reveals the fact that twelve additional permutations have been omitted. They are:

B C A B A B B C A B B C
A B B C B C A B A B B C
A B B C A B B C B C A B

Therefore the list is not exhaustive, as one would expect it to be if the above list were drawn up on purely formal or logical criteria. What is more, the omitted permutations have a common feature. In all of these cases the imbalance between the humours is moderate in character. To take one example: 'BAA' in which the Wind is moderately deranged and the other two only slightly deranged. Small deviation in the ratio of the humours is obviously part of the normal state of things and was not considered as a condition of any significance by the Ayurvedic physicians. The significant permutations are those in which the relative disturbance in the humour is acute. The Ayurvedic physicians use a formal system to predict the way the humours may present themselves and then

Medicine of the Gods 89

abstract from this those cases where morbidity is actually found in the physician's experience.

This point is repeated throughout the following sections of this chapter on the humours. For instance, where only two of the humours are affected (samsarga) and a further one in which one humour is aggravated and another is diminished. The total number of morbid manifestations of the body's humours is sixty-two, which is slightly less than half the number of possible permutations allowable by the matrix.

As a rule, Caraka lays down his classificatory convention and then proceeds in the application of it to specific cases. The fact that there are conventions in use throughout the Caraka Samhitâ is evidence of its rationality. It was mentioned earlier that much of the revolution wrought by Linnaeus in the study of botany and all life-sciences, was not so much due to the empirical aspects of his work, but more to the fact that he devised a workable key or index to his book, a convention by which a particular plant may be located in a handbook. If the reader doubts the significance of this, then try for a moment to identify an unfamiliar bird or flower.

The Range of Ayurvedic experience

Authority is a primary source of knowledge within the epistemological mind-set of Ayurveda. This reliance on authority is often thought to limit the empirical input in the theory. This source even has a technical name in Sanskrit, 'âptopadesha'. Authoritative statements count as a source of empirical knowledge or even as a type of research. There are very few equivalents in ancient Indian medicine of the type of clinical trials common in modern-day medical research where the physician is abstracted in the so-called 'double-blind' experiment. However, the experience of a learned physician should not be overlooked; of all the therapies that are available from an extensive pharmacopoeia, the physician is bound to acquire a knowledge over time as to which remedies have turned out in practice to be the most efficacious. This knowledge is separate from the theoretic postulates of the Ayurvedic system. Every medical practice contains within it an implicit degree of experimentation, which despite its lack of control groups such as those called for in modern experimentation, is nevertheless a valuable source of empirical knowledge if of a more limited variety. This is a tradition that continues into the present-day. Charles Leslie, in his study of the revived Indian pharmaceutical industry, found that Indian companies discover which of the Ayurvedic drugs is worth marketing by the simple expedient of polling several successful Ayurvedic practitioners.[20] One company, `Zandu', supplies drugs free of charge to Ayurvedic hospitals for 'clinical' trials.

The ancient texts record a certain amount of experimentation on patients themselves. There is a very famous anecdote on this score. It is worth noting before relating it that all of the morbid essences are real substances, detectable in the blood, urine and other products of the body. The earlier analysis of the permutation of humours was sufficient to demonstrate that they have to be present or absent in detectable quantities.

> *'Ashoka was taken seriously ill with a rare disease involving the most unpleasant symptoms. Tishyarakshitâ feared that if he died Kunâla would come to the throne and punish her for her immoral behaviour, and so she decided to restore Ashoka to health at all costs. She ordered a search to be made for a sick man with exactly the same symptoms as the king. When one was found he was brought to her in her private apartments, and she killed him on the spot. She cut open his stomach and found that*

it contained an enormous worm. She treated the worm with strong and pungent substances such as pepper and ginger. At last she tried onions and these killed it. So she fed Ashoka with large quantities of onions, which . . . are not normally eaten by high caste people. He eliminated the worm and was cured.'[21]

Although this is unlikely to record an actual experiment, the method it recommends is sound enough. In the Caraka Samhitâ there is a technical term for experiments on a patient; it is 'upashaya'[22], diagnosis after the prescription of certain food articles or other therapies. Caraka concedes that certain ailments are difficult to diagnose by the usual technique of direct observation. The application of some therapies is somewhat experimental. For instance, in a suspected swelling of the vâtika type, he would apply a hot, oily massage in the hope of improving the situation. If his therapy brings relief, he knows his initial diagnosis was correct and it is not one of the other more dangerous types of swelling.[23] There are several other passages that recommend the observation of a patient's reaction to a particular intervention, as a means of inferring the nature of the disease and which incidentally would prove one way or another the efficacy of a particular therapy.

The experience of those outside the medical establishment itself was also important. Physicians were advised to seek the advice of diverse authorities on the effects of herbs and other specifics. Some of the first 'authorities' may even have been animals or their behaviour. The observation of the type of herbs that animals instinctively eat when they are sick is a possible means of identifying medicinal plants. Take for example the fairly commonplace fact that cats eat grass as an emetic when they have a stomach-ache. This is a common observation in ancient cultures, Plutarch mention that the ancient Egyptian medical god 'Thoth' was often depicted as an ibis, a bird that reputed administered its own purges and can detect pure water, facts that were transmuted to the ancient Egyptian.[24] The observation of animal behaviour forms a key part of yoga, a discipline whose history is very closely related to the medical one, many yoga positions are modelled on animal poses - for example, the lion-pose (simhâsana) and the bird-pose (kukkutâsana).[25]

Sushruta recommends that medicinal herbs and plants should be recognized and identified with the help of cowherds, hermits, huntsmen, forest dwellers and those who cull the fruits and edible roots of the forest.[26] Caraka mentions the same source of knowledge, adding that goatherds, shepherds, cowherds and other forest dwellers are aware of the name and form of drugs (oshadhi), and that it is up to the physician to determine the correct application of the drug.[27] This is a very significant admission. It is very probable that a great deal of the Ayurvedic pharmacopoeia was generated by this type of on-the-spot experience. To give a more recent example of the contribution that can be made by lay experts, consider the initial researches of Charles Darwin amongst pigeon fanciers. Through long familiarity with the birds they were able to detect subtle differences between them and exploit those in their selective breeding programmes. The resulting diversity gave Darwin his insight into the origin of all species.

Another important source of Ayurvedic knowledge was the midwife. We have already noted the advanced character of ancient Indian obstetrics and gynaecology and their relation to the philosophical notions of the Sâmkhya system. In common with most other medical traditions, it is unlikely that the male physicians actually assisted in the process of childbirth, except in case of difficulty. The actual business of childbirth was the job of midwives. both Caraka and Sushruta actually tell us this is the case and advise the pregnant woman to heed their advice very closely; an admission of the respect to be granted the experienced midwife.[28]

Another great source of empirical knowledge comes from the physical investigation of the body and under this heading can be included anything from the observation of vital bodily signs, to the analysis of the various bodily products and even dissection. There is a painting in one of the Buddhist cave temples at Ajanta in which the medical monks were learning anatomy by looking at a dead body which had been decomposed by submerging it near a waterfall. Sushruta describes the procedure for the conducting of a dissection in the long section of his compendium dealing with anatomy:

'A dead body selected for this purpose should not be wanting in any of its parts, should not be a person who had lived up to a hundred years (ie, too old) or of one who died from any protracted disease or of poison. The excrement should first be removed from the entrails and the body should be left to decompose in the water of a solitary and still pool, and securely placed in a cage (so that it may not be eaten by fish, nor drift away), after having covered it entirely with the outer sheaths of Muñja grass, Kusha grass, Hemp or with rope etc. After seven days the body would be thoroughly decomposed, when the observer should slowly scrape off the decomposed skin etc with a whisk made of grass-roots, hair, a kusha blade or with a strip of split bamboo; and carefully observe with his own eyes all the various different organs, external and internal, beginning with the skin as described before.'[29]

The inference we can draw from this is that a great deal of real anatomical knowledge displayed in the Ayurvedic texts is based upon these dissections, as well as the keen observation of corpses in various stages of decomposition. Although much of the actual cutting was carried out by assistants, Sushruta instructs that the surgeon must also try things out for himself. In another passage he says that incisions should be practiced on fruit or leather gourds and even the blood vessels of dead animals.[30]

Conclusion

There is sufficient evidence to show that Ayurveda is a rational system which incorporates a great deal of information from correctly observed if sometimes limited experience. It abounds in logical schemas for the classification of the facts of experience. The purpose of these schemas is firstly as an aide-mémoire, allowing a vast array of facts to be mastered. Secondly they offer a way of orientating oneself within a lavish reality. Nobody has ever really denied that these sophisticated classificatory schemas do exist; the feature of them that is slightly less well-known is the fact that they do not overwhelm the data that they are supposed to help master. Ayurvedic theory and experience are linked and there are many examples that have already been given where the facts of experience have clearly been allowed to modify the theoretical model. This dialogue between a theoretical model and its data is a phenomenon highly valued in our own society and one that has come to form the basis of the modern concept of scientific activity.

Appendix

Sushruta's catalogue of meats

1. JANGALA

1.1 Janghâla: Those which have legs

ena	black antelope
harina	antelope
riksha	nilgai
kuranga	tetracere
karâla	musk-deer
kritamala	spotted antelope
sharabha	deer
shvadamshtrâ	mouse-deer
prishata	spotted deer
cârushkara	gazelle?
mrigamâtrikâ	hogdeer

1.2 vishkira: Those which scatter

lâva	quail, partridge
tittiri	partridge
kapiñjala	grey partridge
vartîra)	
vartika)	quail
vârtaka)	
naptrikâ	?
vârtîka	quail
cakora	cakor

kalavinka	sparrow
mayûra	peacock
krakara	quail
upacakra	cakor, duck
kukkuta	cock
sâranga	black & white cuckoo
shatapatra	peacock
kutittiri	partridge
kuruvâhaka	cock?
yavâlaka	?

1.3 Pratuda: Those which peck

kapota	pigeon
pârâvata	pigeon
bhringarâja	drongo with forked tail
parabhrita	cuckoo
koyashtika	lapwing
kulinga	sparrow
grihakulinga	domestic sparrow
gokshvedaka	heron
dindimânavaka	barbet
shatapatraka	woodpecker
mâtrinindaka	?
bhedâshin	?
shuka	parakeet
sârikâ	thrush
valgulî	bat
girishâ	mountain partridge
latvâ	scarlet minivet
lattûshaka	minivet
sugrihâ	tisserin (weaver bird)

khañjarîta	wagtail
hârîta	green pigeon
dâtyûha	poultry

1.4 Guhâshaya: Those which have a lair or den

simha	lion
vyâghra	tiger
vrika	wolf
tarakshu	hyena
riksha	bear
dvîpin	panther
mârjâra	cat
shrigâla	jackal
mrigervâruka	a species of tiger

1.5 Prasaha: Carnivores (those which snatch their food)

kâka	crow
kanka	heron
kurara	osprey
câsha	jay
bhâsa	gypaetus
shashaghâtin	falcon
ulûka	owl
cilli	kite
shyena	eagle
gridhra	vulture

1.6 Parnamriga: Tree dwellers

madgu	?

mûshika	climbing rat
vrikshashâyikâ	squirrel
avakusha	monkey
pûtighâsa	civet
vânara	monkey

1.7 Bileshaya: Burrowing animals

shvâvidh	porcupine
shalyaka	porcupine
godhâ	lizard
shasha	hare
vrishadmsha	cat
lopâka	fox
lomashakarna	?
kadalî	?
mrigapriyaka	snake
ajagara	snake
sarpa	snake
mûshika	rat, mouse
nakula	mongoose
mahâbabhru	mongoose

1.8 Grâmya: Domestic animals

ashva	horse
ashvatara	mule
go	cow
khara	donkey
ushtra	camel
basta	goat
urabhra	sheep
medahpucchaka	fat-tailed sheep

2. ANŪPA

2.1 Kûlacara: Animals which dwell on river banks

gaja	elephant
gavaya	ox
mahisha	buffalo
ruru	barasingha
camara	yak
srimara	wild boar, zebra
rohita	?
varâha	boar
khadgin	rhinoceros
gokarna	cow-eared deer
kâlapucchaka	?
udra	otter
nyanku	deer
aranyagavaya	ox

2.2 Plava: Floating animals

hamsa	goose
sârasa	crane
krauñca	crane
cakravâka	sheldrake
kurara	osprey
kâdamba	teal, duck
kârandava	goose
jîvañjîvaka	Greek partridge
baka	heron, egret
balâkâ	heron, egret
pundarîka	white-eyed pochard

plava	pelican
sharârîmukha	heron
nandîmukha	comb-duck
madgu	cormorant
utkrosha	sea-eagle
kâcâksha	?
mallikâksha	pochard
shuklâksha	pochard
pushkarashâyikâ	lily trother
konâlaka	?
ambukukkutikâ	brook ouzel
megharâva	screamer
shvetavârala	?

2.3 Koshastha: Crustacea

shankha	conch
shankhanaka	?
shukti	oyster
shambûka	conch
bhallûka	cowrie

2.4 Pâdin: Animals with feet

kûrma	tortoise/turtle
kumbhîra	crocodile
karkataka	crab
krishnakarkataka	black crab
shishumâra	crocodile

2.5 Nâdeyâ matsyâh: Fresh-water fish

rohita	carp
pâthîna	sheat fish
pâtalâ	eel
râjîva	mullet
varmi	?
gomatsya	?
krishnamatsya ?	
vâguñjâra	?
murala	?
sahasradamshtra	cat-fish

2.6 Sâmudrâ matsyâh: Marine fish

timi	shark, whale
timingila	large fabulous fish
kulisha	?
pâkamatsya	?
nirula	?
nandivâralaka ?	
makara	fabulous(dolphin)
gargara	Pimelodus gagora
candraka	?
mahâmîna	?
râjîva	mullet

Caraka's catalogue of meats [31]

1. Prasaha: Animals that snatch

go	Cow
khara	donkey
ashvatara	mule
ushtria	camel
ashva	horse
dvîpin	panther
simha	lion
riksha	bear
vânara	monkey
vrika	wolf
vyâghra	tiger
tarakshu	hyena
babhru	mongoose
mârjâra	cat
mûshika	mouse
lopâka	fox
jambuka	jackal
shyena	eagle
vântâda	dog
câsha	jay
vâyasa	crow
shashaghnî	falcon
madhuhâ	buzzard
bhâsa	gypaetus
gridhra	vulture
ulûka	owl
kulingaka	sparrow hawk
dhûmika	owlet

kurara	osprey

2. Bhûmishaya: Burrowing animals

shveta	white snake
shyama	greenish snake
citraprishtha	speckled snake
kâkulîmriga	python
kûrcikâ	hedgehog
cillata	shrew
bheka	frog
godhâ	iguana
shallaka	porcupine
gandaka	gecko
kadalî	marmet
nakula	mongoose
shvâvit	porcupine

3. Anûpa: Marsh animals

shrmara	wild boar
camara	yak
khadga	rhinoceros
mahisha	buffalo
gavaya	ox
gaja	elephant
nyanku	deer
varâha	boar
ruru	deer/barasingha

4. Vârishaya: Aquatic animals

kûrma	turtle
karkataka	crab
matsya	fish
shishumâra	crocodile
timingila	whale
shukti	pearl oyster
shankha	conch
udra	cat fish
kumbhîra	crocodile
culukî	dolphin
makara, etc	crocodile

5. Vâricara: Floating birds

hamsa	goose
krauñca	crane
balâkâ	crane
baka	crane
kârandava	goose
plava	pelican
sharâri	heron
pushkarâhva	lily trother
keshari	comb duck
manitundaka	lapwing
mrinalakantha	snake bird
madgu	cormorant
kâdamba	teal
kâkatunda	river crow
utkrosha	sea eagle/trumpeter
pundarikâksha	pochard
megharâva	screamer
ambukukkuti	water hen

âra	Cobble's owl bird
nandîmukhî	comb duck/flamingo
vâtî	grebe
sumukha	gull
sahacâri	petrel
rohinî	tropical bird
kâmakâlî	frigate
sârasa	crane
raktashirshaka	crane
cakravâka	sheldrake

6. Jângala: Animals of dry terrain

prishata	spotted deer
sharabha	deer
râma	deer
shvadamshtrâ	mouse deer
mrigamâtrikâ	hog deer
shâsha	hare
urana	sheep
kuranga	roe deer
gokarna	mule deer
kottakâraka	barking deer
carushka	gazelle
harina	antelope
ena	black antelope
shambora	deer
kâlapucchaka	black-tailed deer
rishya	nilgai
varapota	deer

7. Vishkira: Gallinaceous birds

lava	quail

vartika	quail
kapiñjala	partridge
cakora	chukor
upacakra	cakor, duck
kukkubha	pheasant
raktavartma	fowl

Vartaka, etc

vartaka	male bustard
vartika	female bustard
barhî	peacock
tittiri	partridge
kukkuta	cock
kanka	heron
sârapada	stork
indrâbha	adjutant
gonarda	partridge
girivartaka	quail
krakara	quail/snipe
avakara	pea-fowl
vârada	spoonbill

3. Pratuda: Pecking birds

shatapatra	woodpecker
bhringarâja	drongo with forked tail/bird of paradise
koyashti	coucal/lapwing
jivañjîvaka	mynah
kairâta	butcher's bird
kokila	koel
atyuha	bulbul

gopâputra	cow-bird
priyâtmaja	babbler
lattâ	scarlet minivet
lattashaka	minivet
babhru	Bengal tree pie
vatahâ	pie
dindimânaka	toucan
jatî	pie
dundubhi	horn-bill
pâkkâra	barbet
lohaprishtha	kingfisher
kulingaka	weaver-bird
kapota	dove
shuka	parakeet
shâranga	parakeet
ciratî	window bird
kanku	parakeet
yashtikâ	sun bird
kalavinka	sparrow
cataka	sparrow
angâracûdaka	wren
pârâvata	pigeon
pândavika	pigeon

Endnotes

1 Aristotle, *The Parts of Animals*, Translated by A L Peck (Loeb: London 1987).

2 Carl von Linné

3 CS.I.27,53-55.

4 Wendy D O'Flaherty, *Hindu Myths* (Harmonsworth: Penguin 1975) page 192.

5 CS.I.15,7.

6 Harley Manuscript 4751, late 12th Century, European, British Library.

7 CS.I.27,8.

8 Commentary on CS.I.27,7-12.

atra ca shâlir haimantikam dhânyam shashtikâdayas' ca graishmakâh vrîhayah shâradâ iti vyavasthâ |

9 CS.I.27,4.

10 Jean Filliozat *The Classical Doctrine of Indian Medicine* English translation by D R Chanana (Munshiram Manoharlal 1964) page 30.

11 Francis Zimmerman *La Jungle et le Fumet des Viandes - Une Thème écologique dans la médicine hindoue* (Gallimard 'Le Seuil' 1982).

12 op cit page 158.

13 Bryan R Wilson (ed) *Rationality* (Oxford: Basil Blackwell 1970) page ix.

14 Bryan R Wilson op cit page xi.

15 CS.I. 25,29

16 CS.I.27 & SS.I.46

17 CS.I.25,29.

18 CS.I.17,41.

19 Richard Fitter, Alistair Fitter and Marjorie Blamey *The Wild Flowers of Britain and Northern Europe* (Collins 1974) q.v..

20 Charles Leslie 'Lecture on the Indigenous Pharmaceutical Industry' (Wellcome Foundation London 28.3.83).

21 E B Cowell & R A Neil (eds) The *Divyâvadana* (Amsterdam: Oriental Press 1970) quoted by A L Basham in Charles leslie (ed) *Asian Medical Systems* (University of Califormia Press 1976).

22 CS.II.1,10; CS.III.4,8.

23 CS.I.18,10.

24 Plutarch *De Iside et Osiride* edited with introduction and translation by J Gwyn Griffiths (University of Wales Press 1970) Chapter 75 page 237.

25 For these and many other examples see: *B K S Iyengar, Light on Yoga*, (Allen & Unwin: London 1968), passim.

26 SS.I.36,10.

27 CS.I.1,120.

28 CS.IV.4,18; translated on page 274 above.

29 SS.III.5,50-56.

30 SS.I.9, passim.

31 CS.I.27,35-52.

Bibliography

Aristotle, *The Generation of Animals*, translated by Peck A L, (Cambridge, Mass : Loeb, 1943).

Ashoka, *The Edicts of*, Nikama N A & McKeon R (University of Chicago Press 1959).

Atharva Veda, translated D Witney (Harvard Oriental Series, 1905)[Reprint,1971].

Avalon A (Sir John Woodroffe), *The Serpent Power* (New York: Dover, 1974).

Bâdarâyana, *Brahmasûtras*, edited by Deussen P, and translated by Johnston C, (Chicago, 1912).

Bapat P V, 'Unidentified Sources of the Vimutti Magga' *Annals of the Bhandarkar Oriental Research Institute* XII 207-11.

Basham A L,'The Practice of Medicine in Ancient India' Leslie C, *Asian Medical Systems*, (Univiversity of California Press 1976).

Beal S, *Buddhist Records of the Western World* (1884).

Beecher H K, *Measurement and Subjective Responses* (Yale UP,1959).

Bhagavad-Gîtâ, Translated by R C Zaehner (OUP 1976).

Bhela Samhitâ, Journal of the Department of Letters, Calcutta University, Vol 8 (Calcutta 1921).

Brihad Aranyaka Upanisad, Translated by S Radhakrishnan (London, Allen & Unwin, 1953).

Burrow T, 'Rajas' *Bulletin of the School of Oriental and African Studies* (XII.645).

Cakrapânidatta, Âyuveda-Dîpikâ on Caraka Samhitâ ed J T Âchârya (Munshiram Manoharlal 1981).

Caraka Samhitâ and Âyurvedadîpikâ of Cakrapânidatta, edited by Kaviraja Harinath Vishârad (Calcutta 1892 and 1914).

Caraka Samhitâ, and Âyurvedadîpikâ of Cakrapânidatta, edited by Vaidya Jâdavaji Trikamji Âchârya, (Bombay 1941, 1981) 4th edition.

Caraka Samhitâ, edited by G S Pândheya (Varanasi 1969).

Caraka Samhitâ, edited by Gangâdhara (Berhampore, 1879).

Caraka Samhitâ, edited by Jîvânanda Vidyasagara (Calcutta, 1877).

Caraka Samhitâ, English translated edition of Avinasha Chandra Kaviratna (Calcutta 1890).

Caraka Samhitâ, Gulabkunverba Âyurvedic Society (Jamnagar, 1949) six volumes.

Caraka, Samhitâ, English translation of the made by R K Sharma & B Dash (Chowkhamba Sanskrit Series 1976).

Chândogya Upanishad, Translated by R C Zaehner (Everyman, London 1977).

Chândogya Upanisada, English translation by T Gelblum, *op cit* .

Chilman Anne M & Thomas Margaret (eds), *Understanding Nursing Care*, 2nd ed (Churchill Livingstone, 1982) .

Chowdhury A K Roy, 'Trepanation in Ancient India' *Asiatic*

Society of Calcutta, Communications Vol 25 (1973).

Christoph Burgel J, 'Secular & Religious Features of Medieval Arab Medicine' published in C Leslie (see below).

Coomaraswami A, *Yaksha* (Washington: 1928).

Copleston R S, *Buddhism*, (London: Longmans, Green & Co 1892).

Dallana, Nibandhasamgraha, edited by Jîvânanda Vidyasagara (Calcutta 1891).

Dallana, Nibandhasamgraha, (Calcutta 1891).

Dandin's Kavyadarsha ed K R Roy (Calcutta 1961).

Dani A H (ed) 'Timargarha and the Gandhara Grave Culture' *Ancient Pakistan* Vol 3 (1967).

Douglas Mary, *Purity & Danger - An Analysis of the Concept of Pollution and Taboo* (RKP 1966).

Dubos R & J, *The White Plague*, (Gollancz, 1953).

Edgerton F, 'The Meaning of Sâmkhya and Yoga', *American Journal of Philology* 45 (1924). 1-46.

Edgerton F, *The Beginnings of Indian Philosophy*, (London, 1965).

Ehrenreich B & English D, *Witches, Midwives and Nurses*, (Compendium: London 1974).

Fa-hsien, The Travels of, translated into English by H A Giles (CUP 1923).

Filliozat J, *The Classical Doctrine of Indian Medicine - Its Origins and Greek Parallels*, English Translation by D R Chanana (Delhi, Munshiram Manoharlal 1964).

Frauwallner E, *History of Indian Philosophy* Vols (Varanasi, Motilal Banarsidas, 1973) English translation by V M Bedekar.

Gangâdhara, *Jalpakalpataru* Commentary on *Caraka Samhitâ*, (1871) BL 14043d 16 Sûtrasthâna chapters 1-5, 57.

Gautama's Nyâyasûtra with Vâtsyayâna-Bhâshya, trans G Jhâ

(Poona 1939).

Gelblum T & Pines S 'Al-Bîrûnî's Arabic Version of Patañjali's Yogasûtra: A Translation and comparison with related texts' *Bulletin of the School of Oriental & African Studies*, Vol XXIX,2,1966 302-25 (YS I); Vol XL, 1977 522-549 (YS.II); Vol XLVI 1983 (YS III); .

Gerow Edwin, *Indian Poetics* (Wiesbaden, 1977).

Gombrich Prof R, 'Sanskrit Manuscripts in the Bodleian Library', Oxford (lecture) .

Government of India Statistical Abstract, 1978: 'Diseases Treated in Hospitals and Dispensaries for 1970'.

Hardy R S, *Manual of Buddhism* (London 1853).

Harley Manuscript 4751, late 12th Century, European, British Library.

Herman A L, *An Introduction to Buddhist Thought* (University Press of America, 1983).

Hippocrates, *Hippocratic Writings* (Penguin 1983).

Hoernle F R (ed) *The Bower Manuscript Facsimile Leaves, Nagari Transcript, Romanized Transliteration and English Translation with notes.* (Calcutta 1893).

Hoernle T, *Studies in the Medicine of Ancient India Osteology* (Oxford 1907).

Horner I B, *The Books of the Discipline* 6 Vols (London : PTS, 1938-66).

Hurry J B, *Imhotep: The Vizier and Physician of King Zoser and Afterwards the Egyptian God of Medicine*, (London: OUP 1926).

I-Tsing, *A Record of the Buddhist Religion as Practiced in India & the Malay Archipelago [AD 677-695]*, Translated into English by Junjiro Takakusu (OUP 1896).

Ishvara Krishna, The Sâmkhya Kârikâ, edited and translated by Sastri S S Suryanarayana, (University of Madras 1935). 2nd ed.

Ishvara Krishna, The Sâmkhya Kârikâ, translated by John Davies (London 1881).

Ishvara Krishna, Sâmkhya Kârikâ translation by G Jha (Poona, 1934).

Iyengar B K S, *Light on Yoga*, (London: Allen & Unwin 1968).

Jalil A, 'Marmas and Acupuncture Points: A Comparative Study.' *Studies in the History of Medicine* 1981 5 18-31.

Johnson E H, *Early Sâmkhya: An Essay on Historical Development According to the Texts* (Royal Asiatic Society 1937).

Jolly J, *Indian Medicine*, Translated from German by C G Kashika (Poona 1951).

Kalyânamalla's Anangaranga, edited and translated in English by N Prasad (Varanasi : Chaukhambha,1983).

Kaulajñânanirnaya, edited by P C Bagchi, translated into English by Michael Magee (Varanasi, 1986).

Keith A B, *The Sâmkhya System* (London, 1918).

Leslie C, 'Lecture on the Indigenous Pharmaceutical Industry' (Wellcome Foundation London 28.3.83).

Leslie C, *Asian Medical Systems* (University of California Press 1977).

Lévi Sylvain, 'Notes sur les Indo-scythes' in *Journal Asiatique*, Nov-Dec 1896.

Lomie I M, 'The Hippocratic Treatise, on the Regimen in Acute Disease', *Sudhoffs Archiv Fur Geschichteder Medizine*, Band 49. 1965.

Lomotte Etienne, *Triate de la Grande Vertu de Sagesse de Nâgârjuna* (1966).

Lovejoy A O, 'The Buddhistic Technical terms upâdâna and upâdisesa' *Journal of the American Oriental Society*, Vol 19 (1897) pages 126-136.

Lowndes Severely J, *Eve's Secrets: A New Perspective on Human Sexuality*, (Bloomsbury: London 1987).

Mâdhava, Sarva-Darshana-Samgraha, translated by Cowell E B & Gough A E (Trubner 1982).

Mâdhavanidâna and its Chief Commentary: Chapter 1-10, Introduction, Translation and Notes by G Meulenbeld (Leiden, Brill, 1974).

Mahâbhârata translated by Buitenen, J A B Van, (University of Chicago Press 1973-).

Mahâbhârata translated by K Gangopâdhyaya and others. (P C Roy, Calcutta 1961).

Mahâbhârata, Critically Edited by V S Sukthanker, S K Belvalkar & P L Vaidya (Poona 1927-).

Mahâbhârata, Roy P C, (Calcutta, 1883-96) in fact by Kesari Mohan Ganguli.

Mahâvagga of the Vinaya Pithaka, translated by I B Horner as *The Books of the Discipline : Mahâvagga* (London 1938-66).

Majjhima-nikâya in *Further Dialogues of the Buddha*, Vol II translated by Lord Chalmers, (SBB, Oxford University Press 1927).

Mannirpalam, 'Tamil Literature' (1930) *Bulletin de la Soc.France de Histoire de la Medicine*' (Janu-Fev 1934).

Manu Smriti, translated by G Bühler as *The Laws of Manu*, SBE Vol XXV (Oxford : Clarendon Press, 1886).

McNeil W, *Plagues & Peoples* (Oxford: Blackwell 1977).

Meulenbeld G J, (ed) *Proceedings of the International Workshop* on *Priorities in the Study of Indian Medicine* (Groninger 1984).

Monier-William M, *Sanskrit-English Dictionary* (Oxford 1899) 2nd edition.

Mukhopadhyaya G N, *History of Indian Medicine*, 3 Vols (Calcutta 1929).

Mukhopadhyaya G, *Surgical Instruments of the Ancient Hindus* (Naahar l977).

Müller R F G, *Altindishe Embryologie* (Leipzig 1955).

Murty K K, 'The Doctrine of Doshas as in Sanskrit Poetics', *Indian Historical Quarterly* 20 .

Nâgârjuna, *Yogashataka*, Translated in French by J Filliozat (L'inst.Fr.d'indologie.62) (Pondichéry 1979).

Norman K R, *Pâli Literature-Including Canonical literature in Prakrit and Sanskrit of all the Hînayâna Schools of Buddhism*, A History of Indian Literature Series (Wiesbaden: Otto Harrassowitz, 1983).

O'Flaherty Wendy D, *Hindu Myths* (Harmondsworth, Penguin 1975).

O'Flaherty Wendy, *Asceticism & Eroticism in the Mythology of Shiva* (OUP, 1973) .

Obeyesekere G, 'The Impact of Âyurvedic Ideas on the Culture and the Individual in Sri Lanka' in *Asian Medical Systems* (University of California Press 1977).

Oldenburg M, *The Buddha: His Life, His Doctrine, His Order*, translated by W Hoey (London 1882).

Pandurangi K T, *The Wealth of Indian MSS in the World* (Bangalore 1978) .

Patañjalî, *Mahâbhâshya*, edited by F Kielhorn, (Bombay 1892).

Patañjali, The Yoga Sûtras of, with Yoga-bhâshya of Vyâsa, translated by Rama Prasada. SBH IV (Allahabad 1924).

Patañjalî, Yoga Sûtra, with Veda Vyâsa Yogabhâshya and Vâcaspâti Mishra's Tattvavaishâradî edited by J Vidyasagara (Calcutta 1874).

Patañjalî, Yogasûtras: with Veda Vyâsa Yogabhâshya and Vâcaspâti Mishra's Tattvavaishâradî (Cambridge, Mass. 1927) edited by Woods J H.

Penzer M N, 'The Romance of Betel Chewing' in Poison Damsels and other Essays in *Folklore and Anthropology* (London 1952).

Pseudo Aristotle, *Secretum Secretorum ad Alexandrum*, Bodl.Ms Ashmole 396, edited by M A Manzalaoui, Early English Text Society 276, (OUP 1977).

Radhakrishnan S & Moore C (eds), *A Sourcebook in Indian Philosophy* (Princetown U P 1973).

Reynolds J E F and Prasad A B (eds), *Martindale's Extra Pharmacopoeia* 28th (Pharmaceutical Press: London 1983).

Rocher L, *The Purânas*, (Wiesbaden, 1986).

Rosu Arion, 'Les Marman et les Art Martiaux Indiens' *Journal Asiatique Tome* CCLXIX 1981.

Roy P C, *History of Indian Chemistry* (London, 1902).

Shankara Mishra, *Commentary on Kanâda Sûtras*, translated by E. Singh (Allahabad 1911).

Sastri D R, *A Short History of Indian Materialism, Sensationalism & Hedonism*, (Calcutta 1930).

Schiefner, *Tibetan Tales*.

Seal B, *The Positive Sciences of the Ancient Hindus* (London 1915).

Sheldon W H, *The Varieties of Human Physique*, with S S Stevens & W B Tucker (New York 1940).

Sing Jee B, *A Short History of Aryan Medical Science* (London).

Sushruta Samhitâ with the commentary Nibandhasamgraha by Dallana, edited by Sengupta Nripendranath and Sengupta Balai Chandra (Pt I, II Calcutta 1938).

Sushruta Samhitâ Kalpasthâna, Translated as *Toxicological Considerations in Ancient Indian Surgery* By Singhal G D & Dwivedi R N (Singhal 1976).

Sushruta Samhitâ with the commentaries of Dhallana and Cakrapânidatta, edited by Sen Vijayaratna and Sen Nisikanta (Calcutta 1901).

Sush*ruta Samhitâ with the commentary of Dhallanâchârya*, edited by Jadavji Trikamji Acharya (Bombay 1915, 3rd edition 1938).

Sushruta Samitâ, English translation of Kaviraj K Bhishagratna (Chowkhamba Sanskrit Series 1963) 2nd edition).

Sushruta, Shârîrasthâna, *Anatomical & Obstetric Considerations in Ancient Indian Surgery* . Translated by Dr G D Singhal & Dr L V Guru (Institute of Medical Sciences, Varanasi 1979 SS.III.1,4.

Sushruta, Samhitâ, Bodl MS Wilson 289 dated 1835-36 .

Sutta-Nipâta, edited by D Anderson (London: PTS, 1913).

Tucci, *Pre-Dinnâga Buddhist Texts on Logic* (Gaekwad's Oriental Series 49, Baroda 1929) .

Vâcaspati Mishra's Tattva-kaumudî, translated by G Jha (Poona 1934).

Vâgbhata I, Âshtânga Hridaya-Samhitâ, English translation from Tibetan by Clause Vogel (Franz Steiner 1965).

Vâgbhata II, Âshthânga-Samgraha, .

Van Buitenen J A B, 'Studies in Sâmkhya' *JAOS* (Vol 77 1957).

Vidyabhusana S C , *A History of Indian Logic - Ancient, Medieval & Modern*, (Motilal Banarsidas 1971). .

Vishnu Purâna, translated by Wilson H H, (Oxford, 1840).

Weiss M, 'A Critical Study of Unmâda in Early Sanskrit Medical Literature.' (University of Penn, Thesis 1977).

Wijesekera O H, *Vedic Gandharva and Buddhist Gandharba*, (University of Ceylon Review III 1945).

Wilson H H, 'On the Medical and Surgical Sciences of the Hindu's,' *Works* Vol III (London 1864), pages 269-276; 380-393.

Winternitz M, *History of Indian Literature* Vol III Part II, English translation S Jha (Motilal Banarsidas 1967). vols I & II, translated by Mrs Ketkar (Calcutta University 1927).

Wise Th A, *Commentary on the Hindu System of Medicine*, (Calcutta 1845).

Zimmer H R, *Hindu Medicine*, (Baltimore 1948).

Zimmerman F, *La Jungle et le Fumet des Viandes - Une Thème écologique dans la médicine hindoue* (Gallimard 'Le Seuil' 1982).

Zinsser H, *Rats Lice & History* (Bantam 1965).

Zvelebil K V, *The Poets of the Powers*, (London: Rider 1973).

Zysk K G, 'Studies in Traditional Indian Medicine in the Pali Canon - Jîvika and âyurveda' *Journal of the International Association for Buddhist Studies* Vol 5 No 1 (1981).

Zysk K, 'Early Vedic Ideas of Disease and Healing with translations and Annotations of Medical Hymns from the Rig Veda and Atharva Veda' (Ph.D Australian National University 1981).

Zysk K, 'Religious Healing in the Veda', *Transactions of the American Philosophical Society* Vol 75 part 7, 1985.

Index

A

acid 16, 32
Agadatantra 33
Air 16
  Type 40
Ajanta 93
Albiruni 30
âlocaka 27
animals 91
  behaviour 75
  medicinal properties 78
anûpa 32
aphrodisiacs 33
Aristotle 74, 78
aryanisation 74
ashmari 69
Ashoka 90
Astringent 16, 32
astrology 44
Atharva Veda 48, 67
Atreya 23
Ayurvedic 57

B

barley 82
bestiary 79
bigotry 12
Bile 21, 24, 25, 32, 37
  black 25
  yellow 21, 25
birds 77
Bitter 16, 32
Blood 21, 25, 26, 55
Blue 21
Bone 21
Bower manuscript 87
Brahma 18
brain 26
Brihad-Âranyaka Upanishad 14
Buddhism 10, 72, 93

C

Cakrapânidatta 81
Caladrius 79
calcium 70

Cancer 66, 71
Caraka 9, 10, 23, 25, 29, 31, 37, 56
  Samhitâ 12
chakras 27
  navel 27
chaulmoogra oil 67
consciousness, seat of 26
constitution 28, 37
  air 40
  fire 39
  water 38
Consumption 48, 57, 71
conventions 89
cooking 24
cough 53
cowherds 92
cysts 65

D

dairy 71
Daksha's sacrifice 71
demon 47
  possession 54

Diabetes 57, 61, 63, 71
Disease 19
  cause of 23
dissection 93
  decomposed 93
dogma 83
dosha 24
dravya 16
dropsy 54

E

earth 16
effect 16
eight limbs 33
eight limbs of Ayurveda 33
elements 25
endemic 46, 74
enlightenment 10
epidemic 46, 74
Epilepsy 57, 68
equipoise 33
European medicine 25
experiments 90, 91
  double-blind 89
  medical research 89
extraction of foreign bodies 33

F

fat 21
fever 52, 53
fiery 39
Fire 16
Fistulas 57

Five Elements 14, 16
flesh 21
fluid 21
forest dwellers 92
Fractures 55
freckles 39

G

gnosticism 19
gulma 66
Guna 19
gynaecology 92

H

Haemorrhage 55
heart 26, 27
  pain 52
heartburn 52
herbs 91
hermits 92
herpes 53
Hippocrates 65
humours 24, 25, 28, 32, 37
  four 25
  function 35
  geography 28
  seasons 28
  taste 32
  three 21, 24, 26
huntsmen 92
Hydnocarpus wightiana 67

I

Indian Dog 78
Indian technique 11

Indra 71
insanity 54
internal medicine 33
Iron-age 74

J

Jângala 32, 74, 75
jaundice 52
Jâyânya 51
Jîvaka 54
Jolly, J 11

K

Kâlikâ Purâna 77
kapha 21, 25, 37
kaphaja 38
Kaumâra bhritya 33
kâyacikitsa 33
kittâ 24, 85
Kshetriyá 51

L

Leprosy 57, 66, 71
leviathan 80
liver 26

M

Mahabharata 17
Mahâbharata 74
makara 80
malaria 52, 74
marrow 21
materia medica 11
matter out of place 25
meat 71, 74, 79
menorrhagia 55
micro-organisms 26
microcosm 18

Ayurveda 123

midwifes 92
millet 81
Mind 19, 42
moon 13, 14

N

natural urges 58
naturalistic 47
nervous diseases 57

O

obstetrics 92
Ojas 21
owl 78

P

Pâcaka 26
Paediatrics 33
pepper 91
pharmacology 11, 92
Phlegm 21, 24, 25, 31, 32, 37
phyto-geography 74
Piles 57, 68
Pitta 21, 25, 26, 37
Pittala 39
plastic surgery 11
Plato 42, 53
Poetics 13
potency 16
prakriti 28, 37
Pungent 15, 32

Q

quality 16

R

rains 81
Rajas 19, 21, 23
Rajasa 42
rañjaka 26
Rápas 52
rasa 13, 24, 26, 81, 85
Rasâyana 33
rationality 89
red 21, 26
Renal Calculus 69
roga 52
Royle 11

S

Saline 15, 32
Salt 16
salvation 10
Sâmkhya 92
sanskritisation 74
sâra 37
Sattva 19, 21, 39, 42
Seasons 82
  Asian 30
  European 31
semen 13, 21
Shâlâkya 33
Shalya 33
shaman 9
sharabha 77, 80
Shiva 71
shlesmala 38
shlesman 25
Shosha 48, 60
siddhis 27
Skin disorders 56

skin graft 11
smell 19
Soma 13
Soul 42
sour 15, 16
Space 16
spirits 13
spleen 26
spoil, to 24
stomach 26
Stones 69
summer 81
surgeon 93
Sushruta 25, 37, 42, 56, 68, 75
  Samhitâ 12
swamp 32
sweet 15, 16, 32
swellings 52
symptoms
  acute 88

T

taboo 10, 26
Takmán 48
Tamas 19, 20, 21, 23
Tamasa 42
Tamil Siddhas 10
Tantra 27, 43
Taraktogenos
  kurzii 67
taste 14, 15, 31, 85
  six 14, 15
temperament 37, 42
Tetanus 53

timi *80*
timingila *80*
Tissues 21
Tonics *33*
Toxicology *33*
Treatment of head and neck *33*
trepanning *54*
Tuberculosis 48, 57, 60
Tumours 57, 65

U

udara *54*
Unctuous *38*
unicorn *79*
Urinary calculi *57*

urine *61, 62*
retention 55

V

Vâgbhata *29*
Vâjikarana *33*
vâta *21, 37*
vataja *40*
vâyu *25*
Vedas *13*, 18, *45, 46, 47*
and desease 47
Vimânasthâna *37*
vipâka *16*
vîrya *16*

W

waste *24*

wasting 53
Water *16, 38*
Western physicians *11*
Wilson, H H *11*
Wind *21, 24, 25, 31, 32, 37*
winter *81*
worms 54, *91*

Y

Yákshma 48
Yoga *27, 92*

Z

Zandu *90*
zoology *78*
Zysk *47*

Also in this Series.

The Siddha Quest for Immortality.

By Professor Kamil Zvelebil.

One of the foremost experts on Tamil culture and author of *Poets of the Powers*.

.

'Siddha' means magical or supernatural power. It is also the name taken by adherents of a 'tantrik' and ecstatic cult, found now mainly in South India. This new book is written in clear and non technical language and yet explains in much greater detail the hitherto secret and esoteric elements of the Siddha cult. Topics covered include:

.

On Siddhas Medicine.

The Ideological Basis of Siddhas Quest of Immortality.

Basic Tenets of Siddhas Medicine.

Diseases and Their Cure.

Yoga in Siddhas Tradition.

Daily Regime.

Siddhas Alchemy.

Rejuvenation, Longevity, and 'Immortality'.

Doctrines and Traditions of the Siddhas.

Tantrik Siddhas and Siddhas Attitudes to Sex.

Siddhas Poetry and Other Texts.

.

ISBN 1 869928 431.

Price £14.99

Reserve your copy now from .

Mandrake *of Oxford,*.

PO Box 250.

Oxford, OX1 1AP (UK) tel: +(01865) 243671.

www.mandrake.uk.net